NEW DEVELOPMENTS IN MEDICAL RESEARCH

DIVERTICULITIS

DIAGNOSIS AND TREATMENT

NEW DEVELOPMENTS IN MEDICAL RESEARCH

Additional books and e-books in this series can be found on Nova's website under the Series tab.

NEW DEVELOPMENTS IN MEDICAL RESEARCH

DIVERTICULITIS

DIAGNOSIS AND TREATMENT

DR. SHAMS-UL-BARI

AND

PROF. AJAZ A. MALIK

EDITORS

nova
Medicine & Health
New York

Library of Congress Cataloging-in-Publication Data

ISBN: 978-1-53618-081-7
Names: Bari, Shams ul-, editor. | Malik, Ajaz Ahmad, editor.
Title: Diverticulitis : diagnosis and treatment / [edited by] Shams-ul-Bari, Ajaz A. Malik.
Description: Hauppauge : Nova Science Publishers, 2020. | Series: New developments in medical research | Includes bibliographical references and index. |
Identifiers: LCCN 2020024290 (print) | LCCN 2020024291 (ebook) | ISBN 9781536180817 (paperback) | ISBN 9781536180824 (adobe pdf)
Subjects: LCSH: Diverticulitis--Diagnosis. | Diverticulitis--Treatment.
Classification: LCC RC862.D6 D59 2020 (print) | LCC RC862.D6 (ebook) | DDC 616.3/44--dc23
LC record available at https://lccn.loc.gov/2020024290
LC ebook record available at https://lccn.loc.gov/2020024291

Published by Nova Science Publishers, Inc. † New York

DEDICATION

WE DEDICATE THIS BOOK TO OUR PARENTS AND FAMILY MEMBERS, WITHOUT WHOSE SUPPORT AND BLESSINGS THIS VENUTURE WOULD NOT HAVE BEEN POSSIBLE

CONTENTS

PREFACE

Diverticular disease is a benign acquired condition of colon which can cause significant symptoms, impair quality of life and on occasion can be fatal if left untreated. Diverticular disease is the most common structural abnormality of the colon and fifth most costly gastrointestinal disorder in the Western world. Diverticular disease is a disease of western population. Over past 30 years the incidence has increased significantly. Migrant studies have confirmed an increase in incidence when population moves to western country. The prevalence of diverticulosis is age dependent and increases from less than 20% at 40 to 60% at 60 years. The distribution of the disease also varies geographically with western population having prevalence rates of 5-45% and Asian population having prevalence rates of 13-25%. In western population disease predominantly involves left sided colon while as in Asian population right sided colon is more frequently involved. The distribution also varies with race. While both blacks and whites have a higher prevalence of left sided diverticular disease, the distribution of diverticula in ascending colon and hepatic flexure is higher in black as compared to whites. The overall prevalence has increased in both western and Asian population due to adoption of western lifestyle. In the western and industrialized world, diverticular disease of colon is a significant contributor of health care costs and is an important cause of recurrent outpatient visits and hospital admissions.

There are several risk factors that have been associated with diverticular disease .These include high dietary intake of red meat, low fiber intake, lack of vigorous activity, high Body mass index (BMI) and smoking. Diverticular disease of colon is usually asymptomatic in about 70-80%. In symptomatic patients it can present either as bleeding or inflammation (diverticulitis), which could be either simple or complicated due to perforation, peritonitis, obstruction, intraperitoneal abscess and fistula formation. Thc prcscnting clinical features of diverticulitis vary according to the location and severity of the underlying inflammatory process. The left lower quadrant pain is the most common symptom of the patients and may be seen in around 70% patients and is the most common reason for which patients report to the hospital. Patients with irritable bowel syndrome or painful colonic spasm may present with abdominal complaints similar to mild acute diverticulitis and need to be differentiated from true diverticulitis. Many patients remain asymptomatic and colonic diverticula remain undetected until these patients either develop an acute attack or are diagnosed incidentally during colonic investigations. On Physical examination the most common finding will be the tenderness or a mass in the left lower quadrant of the abdomen due to pericolic inflammation or abscess formation. A tender abdominal mass is present in 20% cases and its presence indicates a poor prognosis .Abdominal distension has been reported in about two-thirds of the patients.

Most of the patients are diagnosed on the basis of the history and clinical presentation. Computed tomography of abdomen is the most valuable investigation for diagnosis of diverticulitis and its complications. Colonoscopy and contrast radiography is avoided when acute diverticulitis is suspected as risk of perforation is high. It should be done 6-8 weeks after the inflammation has subsided. In absence of systemic signs and symptoms most of the patients of diverticulitis will respond to antibiotics, analgesics and bowel rest as an outdoor treatment. Antibiotics to be instituted should cover both the Gram negative and anaerobic bacteria. The patients with systemic signs and symptoms of diverticulitis need to be hospitalized. Nothing should be given orally and patients should be put on nasogastric suction, i/v fluids, broad spectrum antibiotics and opioid analgesics given as and when needed.

Approximately, 10-20% patients may need surgical intervention. Wide spectrum of disease is encountered, hence the treatment should be tailored according to patient's presentation. There has been an increasing trend in recent years to treat even patients having recurrent attacks of diverticulitis conservatively, although only in absence of any complications. However, indications of surgery in an elective setting in absence of any complications are still controversial. Sound clinical judgment is required to decide when to intervene. Septic complications such as abscess formation, free perforation and peritonitis are the most common complications which need surgical intervention. Abscess can be drained adequately by placing a percutaneous drain. Surgical options include Hartmann resection, sigmoid resection with primary anastomosis, sigmoid resection with primary anastomosis with proximal diversion and on table lavage with primary anastomosis or laparoscopic lavage without resection. Hartmann procedure is the most common procedure performed for perforated diverticulitis with disadvantage of permanent stoma in about one third of patients. However, emergency procedures have been associated with overall higher morbidity and mortality.

Both laparoscopic and open surgical approaches have been performed to deal with such entities. However the quality of surgery is more important than whether the operation is performed by open or by minimal access approach. With the increasing experience in laparoscopy, minimally invasive surgery is being widely employed in emergency situations such as generalized peritonitis due to diverticulitis. Multiple prospective studies and retrospective analysis in colorectal surgery have confirmed that the laparoscopic approach provided better outcome than the open approach .The advantages of laparoscopy are less postoperative pain, improved respiratory function, short hospital stay and lowered postoperative morbidities. The laparoscopic approach has been performed in all types of procedures related to complicated diverticular disease, such as Hartman procedure, sigmoid resection with primary anastomosis (RPA) and reversal of Hartman procedure. Laparoscopic lavage drainage, a previously unknown technique for the management of purulent peritonitis is also gaining acceptance and has provided new therapeutic approach in the management of complicated diverticulitis.

The book presents an up to date review of the medical and surgical management of diverticulitis. The publication comprises of various topics discussing the background, epidemiology, etiology, pathogenesis, presentation, treatment and recent advances in the management of diverticulitis.

The book will be of academic interest to all the students of medicine both undergraduates and post graduates and can be used as a reference book by teachers, academicians and researchers. The main benefit of reading this book is that since this disease entity is common all over the world and its incidence is increasing and is a significant contributor of health care costs, all the relevant and latest information regarding this disease has been published in a comprehensive form which will be helpful to the researchers, students and medical professional dealing with delivery of health care facilities.

Dr Shams ul Bari

Prof. Ajaz A Malik

In: Diverticulitis: Diagnosis and Treatment ISBN: 978-1-53618-081-7
Editors: Shams-ul-Bari et al.

Chapter 1

DIVERTICULAR DISEASE OF COLON: ETIOPATHOGENESIS AND PRESENTATION

Ajaz Ahmad Malik*
Department of General and Minimal Access Surgery,
SKIMS Srinagar, Jammu and Kashmir, India

ABSTRACT

With the increase in the prevalence of the diverticular disease in the western society, the management of the disease is becoming a financial burden in the systems with limited resources. Little evidence exists that the change in lifestyle may decrease the prevalence of the disease. There are several risk factors that have been associated with diverticular disease. These include high dietary intake of red meat, low fiber intake, lack of vigorous activity, high BMI (>25 kg/m^2) and smoking. Fortunately enough, the diverticular disease is mostly asymptomatic. The presenting clinical features of diverticulitis vary according to the location and severity of the underlying inflammatory process. The left lower quadrant pain is the most common symptom of the patients and may be seen in around 70%, hence being the most common reason for which patients report to the hospital. On physical examination, the most common finding will be the tenderness

* Corresponding Author's Email: ajazamalik@rediffmail.com.

or a mass in the left lower quadrant of the abdomen due to pericolic inflammation or abscess formation. Abdominal distension has been reported in about two-thirds of the patients.

Majority of the patients are diagnosed on the basis of history and physical examination. Certain surgical conditions such as appendicitis, perforated duodenal ulcer and perforated colon cancer have same presentation and need to be excluded. Computed tomography of abdomen is the investigation of choice for diagnosis of diverticulitis and its complications. Most of the cases can be treated with bowel rest and antibiotics while as 10-20% patients may need surgical intervention. Abscess can be drained adequately by placing a percutaneous drain. However the quality of surgery is more important than whether the operation is performed by open or by minimal access approach. Wide spectrum of disease is encountered, hence the treatment should be tailored according to patient's presentation. Sound clinical judgment is required to decide when to intervene.

Introduction

In the western and industrialized world, diverticular disease of colon is a significant contributor of health care costs and also an important cause of recurrent outpatient visits and hospital admissions. Diverticular disease is a benign acquired condition of colon which can cause significant symptoms, impair quality of life and on occasion can be fatal if left untreated. Contrary to western population, in whom diverticula occur predominantly on the left side, mainly sigmoid colon, in Asian population right sided diverticula are more common. Diverticular disease is the most common structural abnormality of the colon and fifth most costly gastrointestinal disorder in the western world [1, 2].

History

Littre in 1700 initially described diverticular disease as saccular out-pouching of the colon [3]. The credit of the first clear and detailed description of the pathogenesis of diverticulitis and complications of diverticular disease goes to Cruveilhier [4]. Graser in 1899 introduced the term "peri-diverticulitis" and suggested that diverticular disease was caused by herniation of colonic mucosa through the weak areas from where vasa recta penetrated the colonic wall [5]. In 1904, Edwin Beer first described the mechanism of diverticulitis ascribing the lodging of hard fecal matter in diverticula as the cause of diverticulitis and subsequently leading to abscess and fistula formation [6]. In 1907, Moynihan, while reporting a case of peri-diverticulitis, underlined the difficulties in differentiating diverticular disease from malignancy [7]. Quervain E et al. and Case JT et al. in 1914 were first to demonstrate colonic diverticula on X-rays [8, 9].

DEFINITIONS

A diverticulum is a sac like protrusion from colon wall. They can be a true or false diverticula. A true diverticulum (pleural: diverticula) is composed of all the layers of colonic wall, whereas a pseudo-diverticulum is herniation of mucosa through muscular layer. Diverticulosis is presence of diverticula which is usually asymptomatic. Diverticular disease is an umbrella term which presents as clinically significant complicated diverticulosis or symptomatic uncomplicated disease. Diverticulitis is an inflammation of diverticula which can be acute or chronic and complicated or uncomplicated. Segmental colitis associated with diverticula is an inflammation of inter diverticular mucosa without involvement of diverticular orifices. Smoldering diverticular disease is characterized by the presence of persistent pain in the absence of clinically overt colitis. It is suspected when increased wall thickness is seen on computed tomography without inflammatory changes.

EPIDEMIOLOGY

Diverticular disease is a disease of western population. Over past 30 years the incidence has increased significantly [10, 11]. Migrant studies have confirmed an increase in incidence when population moves to a western country. The prevalence of diverticulosis is age dependent and increases from <20% at 40 to 60% at 60 years [12, 13]. The distribution also varies geographically with western population having prevalence rates of 5-45% and Asian population having prevalence rates of 13-25%. In western population, disease predominantly involves left sided colon while as in Asian population right sided diverticulosis is more frequently seen [14, 15]. The presence of right-sided diverticula is considered a distinct disease from left-sided diverticulosis, and is thought to be largely due to genetic predispositions. The distribution also varies with race. While both blacks and whites have a higher prevalence of left sided diverticula, the distribution of diverticula in ascending colon and hepatic flexure is higher in black as compared to whites (20 v/s 5.8%). The overall prevalence has increased in both western and Asian population probably due to adoption of western lifestyle. Industrialization and development has been shown to increase rates of diverticulosis. The prevalence of diverticula in colon increases substantially with age. Prevalence of diverticulosis is only 1 to 2% in patients less than 30 years of age [16, 17]. It increases to 50 to 66% in patients older than age 80 years [18]. Approximately 10 to 25% of patients with diverticulosis will develop diverticulitis [19, 20]. The prevalence of the disease in men is approximately equal to that of women. McConnell et al. reported that stricture and obstruction is more frequent in woman while as diverticular bleeding occurs more commonly in men [21].

Risk Factors

There are several lifestyle factors which have been associated with diverticular disease such as high dietary intake of red meat, low fiber intake, lack of vigorous activity, high BMI (>25 kg/m^2) and smoking. Disease is less common in Asia and Africa where diet contains lot of natural fiber, although in Southeast Asia, right sided diverticular disease is more common with manifestations early in life. The etiology behind this variation is unknown, however both diet and elastin/collagen differences have been suggested to play a role [19]. Many genetic, environmental and epidemiological factors have been incriminated as risk factors.

Dietary Factors

High fat and red meat intake have been found to increase the risk of symptomatic diverticular disease whereas vegetarian diet and high fiber has been associated with decrease in the incidence of symptomatic diverticulosis as they decrease the inflammation and alter intestinal micro-biota. Fiber is thought to decrease intra-colonic pressures, decrease transit times, increase weight and volume of stool and contribute to more frequent bowel movements. However the role of fiber in development of diverticular disease or reducing symptoms in uncomplicated disease is still debatable [18, 19].

1) Seeds and Nuts: Consumption of Seeds, corn, popcorn and nuts, as was believed before, are not associated with increased risk of diverticulosis, diverticulitis or bleeding [18, 19].
2) Physical activity: Vigorous activity such as jogging and running have been associated with decreased risk of diverticulitis and diverticular bleeding [20, 21].
3) Obesity: Decreased physical activity and the presence of obesity have been shown to increase the risk of diverticular disease by many researchers. Aldoori and colleagues [21] conducted a review over a period of 4 years to study the relation between the amount of physical activity and the diverticular disease and concluded that physical activity is inversely related to the development of diverticular disease, even when other factors such as fiber intake are controlled. Obesity has also been found to increase the risk of both diverticulitis and diverticular bleeding [21-23].
4) Smoking: It has been suggested that smoking may increase the risk of complications of diverticular disease as higher incidence of diverticulitis has been reported in smokers as compared to non-

smokers. However, several recent studies have failed to show a link between smoking and diverticular bleeding [24, 25].

5) Caffeine and alcohol ingestion: It has been suggested that caffeine has a role to play in the development of diverticular disease as it stimulates small bowel secretions and may affect colonic transit time. Similarly some researchers have also suggested that alcohol consumption may have a role in the pathogenesis of diverticular disease. However other researchers have not found any association between alcohol and caffeine consumption with diverticular disease [22, 26, 27].
6) Medications: Medications such as statins have been shown to decrease the risk of diverticular perforation whereas non- steroidal anti- inflammatory drugs, opiates and steroids have shown to increase the risk [28-31].
7) Vitamin D: Increased vitamin D levels have been shown to decrease risk of hospitalization in diverticulitis [32].
8) Inflammation: Evidence suggests that inflammation may also play a role in the early pathogenesis of the diverticular disease [33]. Positive response to treatments with anti-inflammatory drugs such as mesalazine and 5-ASA suggest that inflammation may play a larger role in pathogenesis of diverticular disease [34, 35].
9) Role of colonic flora: The role of micro-flora in the development and progression of diverticular disease has been the topic of debate in recent times. It has been suggested that alteration in micro-flora of colon may predispose patients to micro-perforation and low-level inflammation by impairing mucosal barrier function and up-regulating inflammatory cytokine release [36]. In a randomized study by Tursei et al. [37], 90 patients with symptomatic diverticular disease were divided into three groups. One group received mesalazine only, the other group received Lactobacillus casei while as the third group received both. The study found the combination treatment to be superior in preventing symptom recurrence [37]. A similar study comparing the results of balsalazide, an amino salicylate compound, and a complex of probiotics, found that the

combination of balsalazide and probiotics was associated with better outcome [38].

10) Urbanization: There is an evidence which suggests that urbanization has led to increase in the incidence of disease.
11) Age: Age is a major risk factor for diverticulosis. Diverticulosis is uncommon before age of 40, and incidence increases after that. About one-third of all Americans develop diverticulosis by age of 60, and two-thirds will have it by age 85 years.
12) Environmental and genetic risk factors are also being studied.

PATHOGENESIS

Arfwidsson et al. performed manometry on subjects with and without sigmoid diverticula, and showed higher luminal pressures in those with diverticular disease [39]. Studies have shown that myo-electrical patterns differ in patients with diverticular disease compared to healthy subjects and have also reported hyper motility in descending and sigmoid colon in patients with diverticular disease. Patients with diverticulosis show slow wave motility patterns of 12 to 18 cycles per minute as compared to 3 cycles per minute pattern observed in irritable bowel syndrome [40-42]. Increased amounts of disorganization and retrograde propagation of propulsions has been observed in patients with diverticular disease [43]. The role of chemical mediators on colonic motility in diverticular disease has also been investigated. It has been observed that the diverticular colon is more strongly innervated by cholinergic nerves than the normal colon and that non-adrenergic, non-cholinergic inhibitory nerves act to a lesser extent in the diverticular colon [44]. A study by Milner and colleagues revealed that vasoactive intestinal polypeptide (VIP) content of the mucosa and whole wall was increased in diverticular disease [43]. Serotonin is known to be a primary trigger of gut motility and its role in diverticular disease has also been investigated. It has been found that although serotonin levels are comparable in patients with and without diverticular disease, but there is a significant attenuation of 5-HT transporter in patients with recent attack of diverticulitis [44-46].

The colonic wall has specific weak points at the areas where vasa-recta enter the circular muscle layer. When the pressure inside the lumen increases due to abnormal colonic motility associated with exaggerated segmentation contractions, dividing the colon into chambers or compartments, the mucosa and submucosa of colon herniates through these points of weakness, resulting into diverticula formation. This process is called segmentation. This effect could be further increased by lack of fiber in the diet [47]. Since the sigmoid colon has the smallest diameter, it is the segment of highest pressure according to the Laplace's law. It has been proved by Painter and others that the basal pressure of the sigmoid colon is a few millimeters of mercury above atmospheric pressure in both patients with and without diverticular disease. However, in patients with symptomatic diverticular disease, high pressure waves that normally have an amplitude of 10 mm Hg can have amplitudes as high as 90 mm Hg or more [48, 49]. In some cases, the arteriole that penetrates the wall is displaced over dome of diverticulum resulting in torrential bleeding.

Morphological Features

In contrast to the small intestine and rectum, the muscularis propria of colon wall is composed of only one complete inner circular muscular layer while as the outer longitudinal layer is assembled in the three taeniae coli. One of the taeniae coli is located on the mesenteric aspect of the colon and is known as taenia mesentericus while the other two are located on the medial and lateral aspects of the bowel wall and are respectively known as taenia omentalis and taenia libra [50]. The colonic wall is weakest at the points between the mesenteric and anti-mesenteric taeniae, where the vasa recta penetrate the muscle as there is atrophy of circular muscle at these sites. It is at these sites that mucosa and submucosa herniate and form diverticula. Hernia formation occurs rarely through the taeniae.

Diverticular disease is associated with change in the histological structure of the colon. Increase in connective tissue component occurs due to repeated intermittent distension of the colon [51]. It is proposed that western diet with its lower fecal load intermittently distends the bowel wall and results in elastin deposition. The deposition of elastin and collagen in the colonic wall is increasingly being recognized. The thickened and contracted appearance of the diverticulum affected colon can be explained by elastosis. The taenia shorten and the colon looks like concertina. Decrease in caliber occurs due to projection of thickened circular muscular folds into the lumen. Due to chronic inflammation mesocolon is also shortened. One study showed that in patients with diverticulitis, there is decrease in the ratio of type 1 and type 111 collagen. The expression of matrix metalloproteinase is also reduced significantly [52]. Diverticular disease has a common association with connective tissue disorders such as Ehlers-Danlos syndrome [53].

CLINICAL FEATURES

Diverticular disease of colon is usually asymptomatic in about 70-80%. In symptomatic patients it can present either as bleeding or inflammation (diverticulitis), which could be either simple or complicated due to perforation, peritonitis, obstruction, abscess formation or fistula (Figure 1). The presenting clinical features of diverticulitis vary according to the location and severity of the underlying inflammatory process [54, 55]. Patients with true acute diverticulitis usually present with signs and symptoms of ongoing inflammation such as progressive localized pain, anorexia, fever and leukocytosis. Patients with irritable bowel syndrome or painful colonic spasm may present with abdominal complaints similar to mild acute diverticulitis and need to differentiate from true diverticulitis. Surprisingly, the clinical manifestations of diverticular disease are relatively infrequent given the high incidence of the disease. Many patients remain asymptomatic and colonic diverticula remain undetected until these patients either develop an acute attack or are diagnosed incidentally during colonic investigations.

Symptomatic acute attack typically presents as pain in left iliac fossa which is usually constant and often persisting for several days. However, if the sigmoid colon is redundant, pain can also be present in right iliac fossa or supra-pubic region. The left lower quadrant pain may be seen in around 70% patients and is the most common reason for which patients report to the hospital. The pain is usually present several days before the patients report to the clinician, which helps us to differentiate true diverticulitis from other surgical emergencies such as appendicitis, perforated colon cancer and perforated peptic ulcers. Less than 17% patients report to hospital within 24 hours after the start of symptoms. History of previous episodes of pain is seen in about 50% of the patients. In about 20-60% of patients nausea and vomiting can occur either due to obstruction or ileus due to peritoneal irritation. Some patients also present with fever. Hypotension and shock is rare and is usually seen in patients with perforation peritonitis. Patients may also present with altered bowel habits, with constipation in 50% and diarrhea in 25%. Urinary tract symptoms due to bladder irritation, such as dysuria, urgency and increased frequency is seen in 15% patients [56, 57].

On physical examination, the most common finding will be the tenderness or a mass due to pericolic inflammation or abscess. Abdominal distension has been reported in about two-thirds of the patients [58, 59]. Tenderness is usually localized to left lower quadrant. Occasionally tenderness may be felt in right lower quadrant, which may be either due to right sided diverticulitis or inflammation of redundant loop of sigmoid colon. Such patients are initially diagnosed as cases of acute appendicitis and diagnosis becomes clear on laparotomy. A tender abdominal mass is present in 20% cases and its presence indicates a poor prognosis. A rectal mass could be felt on digital rectal examination if there is a distal sigmoid abscess.

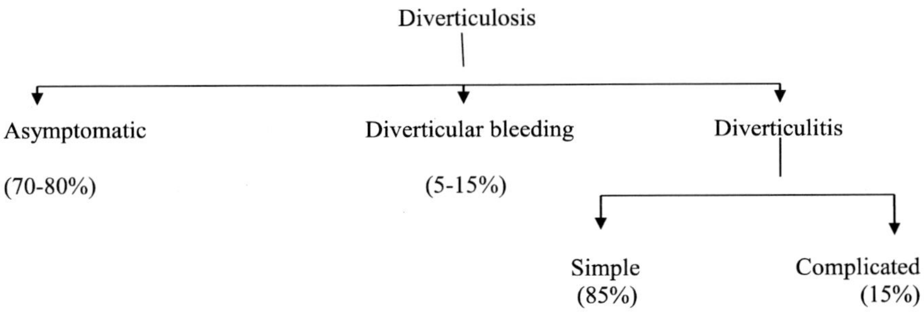

Figure 1. Natural history of disease.

Unusual Extra-Abdominal Presentations

Multiple organ systems may be involved in diverticular disease having unusual presentation especially in case of patients who are immuno-compromised (Table 1). Computed tomography (CT) scans may play a major role in delineating the extent of disease.

Table 1. Extra-abdominal presentations of diverticular disease

Dermatological	Pyoderma gangrenosum
Soft tissue	Thigh Abscess Necrotizing fasciitis
Urinary	Urethral obstruction Colo-urethral fistula
Orthopedic	Osteomyelitis Arthritis
Gynecological	Colouterine fistula Ovarian tumor/abscess
Genital	Epididymitis Pneumoscrotum
Neurological	Colo-epidural fistula
Vascular	Femoral vein thrombosis Mesenteric vein thrombosis Pylebhlebitis Colovenous fistula
Perineal	Fournier's gangrene Complex anal fistula.

Complications of Diverticulitis

Most of the patients having diverticula are asymptomatic. Symptomatic complications are seen in only 10 to 30%. Around 1 to 25% patients present with features of peritonitis. Major impact on outcome in acute phase is usually determined by the degree of infection present. Inflammatory type has lower mortality than perforated ones. Following are the various presentations of complicated diverticulitis [60].

1) Diverticular abscess: It is the most common complication and may occur in 15-20% of patients and has symptoms similar to acute diverticulitis. It occurs when center of phlegmon becomes necrotic. The abscess may present as an abdominal mass, fever and refractory pain. In a patient who initially presents with uncomplicated diverticulitis and whose pain doesn't subside with medications or fever persists even after 3 days of antibiotic therapy, diverticular abscess should be suspected. Sigmoid mesocolon is the most common site for diverticular abscess. Rarely, these patients may present as liver abscess.
2) Obstruction: Obstruction may occur due to luminal narrowing resulting from peri-colic stranding or due to abscess formation. In chronic cases, obstruction can occur due to stricture formation. Often the obstruction is incomplete. There can be associated small gut obstruction as well if a loop of small bowel is incorporated in peri-colic inflammatory mass or due to ileus caused by local irritation. The clinical presentation of the patient depends on level of obstruction.
3) Perforation and peritonitis: About 1-2% of patients present with perforation either due to inflamed diverticula or ruptured abscess leading to fecal or purulent peritonitis respectively. In such cases morbidity is high and signs and symptoms are consistent with peritonitis due to any other cause. Mortality rates range from 12-36% and is most often affected by patient's underlying fitness for surgery.

4) Bleeding: Severe hemorrhage from diverticular disease is rare. The biggest challenge is to differentiate diverticular bleeding from other causes as the disease is so prevalent. In the elderly population the most common cause of rectal bleeding is angiodysplasias and together with diverticular disease, it accounts for 90% of severe lower gastrointestinal hemorrhage. Diverticular bleeding is most common in patients who take non-steroidal anti-inflammatory drugs (NSAIDs) and presents as abrupt passage of large amount of bright or dark red blood per rectum associated with lower abdominal pain. CT angiography is most useful diagnostic tool for localizing site of bleeding when the bleeding exceeds 0.5ml/min. However technetium-99m-labeled sulfur colloid scan is more sensitive test but the accuracy in localizing the site of bleeding is not as good as CT angiography. In 70-80% of patients, diverticular bleeding ceases spontaneously, however the rate of re-bleeding is quite high.
5) Fistula: Fistula formation can occur between colon and any other adjacent organ e.g., bladder, vagina, skin following inflammation from acute diverticulitis. Colovesical fistula is most common and presents with pneumaturia, faecaluria or dysuria. Patients with colovaginal fistula present with passage of faeces or flatus from vaginal opening. Colocutaneous fistula is rare. Malignancy and Crohn's disease should be excluded while evaluating these patients.

Differential Diagnosis

While evaluating patients of diverticular disease, certain disorders with similar presentation need to be ruled out, which include appendicitis, bowel obstruction, ischemic colitis, inflammatory bowel disease, irritable bowel syndrome, urinary tract infection, kidney stones, pyelonephritis, colorectal and gynecological malignancies.

Diagnosis

Most of the patients are diagnosed on the basis of their clinical presentation. Since certain surgical conditions such as appendicitis, perforated duodenal ulcer and perforated colon cancer have same presentation, various investigations are required to reach to the diagnosis. The goal of evaluation is (a) to establish a diagnosis (b) to rule out other differentials. Evaluation begins with history and physical examination as discussed, followed by laboratory tests which includes complete blood count, electrolytes, uric acid level, and pregnancy test in women of child bearing age. In patients with suspected perforation and peritonitis, LFT, serum amylase and lipase levels should be done to rule out other differentials. Mild leukocytosis is a common laboratory finding and a leukocyte count of more than 15000/cu.mm are more likely to have an intra-abdominal abscess [58, 59]. Urine examination may reveal an increased number of leukocytes in urine if the inflammatory process is adjacent to ureter or bladder. The presence of bacteria in urine, particularly colonic flora is a strong indication of presence of fistula between the inflamed colon and the urinary tract. Stool may be positive for occult blood test. In a patient presenting with diarrhea, stool examination for giardia, salmonella, and shigella should be done.

Imaging

Following imaging tests should be utilized to reach to diagnosis.

X-Ray Abdomen

Routine abdominal and chest X-rays are usually unremarkable, although around 30% patients may have some abnormality on radiography. Free gas under diaphragm is an unusual finding in diverticulitis. Retroperitoneal air or a mass effect secondary to large para-colic abscess is occasionally seen in patients with diverticulitis. X-ray abdomen can be performed to rule out complications such as intestinal obstruction and pneumoperitoneum due to perforated viscera [52-56].

Abdominal Ultrasonography

Ultrasonography is a cheap and easily available tool of investigation and avoids radiation exposure. However it is operator dependent and cannot exclude other causes. Features suggestive of acute diverticulitis on ultrasonography include hypo echoic area of peridiverticular reaction, bowel thickening of >4 mm at point of maximum tenderness and presence of diverticula in surrounding segment. Complications of diverticulitis can also be seen by ultrasound.

Colonoscopy and Contrast Radiography

Colonoscopy and contrast radiography is avoided when acute diverticulitis is suspected as risk of perforation is high, due to increased intraluminal pressure caused by injection of contrast material or insufflation of air that may lead to free rupture of a previously localized pericolic abscess or phlegmon. These two investigations had a very important diagnostic role before the availability of computed tomography, but are rarely used nowadays during active diverticulitis due to above reasons. However, both contrast study and colonoscopy can be performed to rule out other colonic conditions usually 6-8 weeks after the inflammation has subsided. In case of major GI bleeding, colonoscopy is performed to rule out malignancy, polyps or site of diverticular bleeding. Contrast study will reveal the typical saw toothed appearance of peridiverticular state. Such spastic strictures are relaxed by probanthin and this helps us to differentiate it from true obstruction due to neoplasm. In any suspected case of diverticulitis, entire colon should be evaluated to know the extent of disease. Sometimes the diverticular inflammation can lead to severe stricture formation that mimics colon cancer. In such a situation, multiple biopsies are recommended to rule out malignancy.

On colonoscopy, diverticulum is seen as a mucosal out pouching (Figure 2). In acute inflammation colonoscopy can be performed with extreme caution, as there are increased chances of perforation and less chances of completion of the procedure. In general, it should be delayed till the inflammation has subsided.

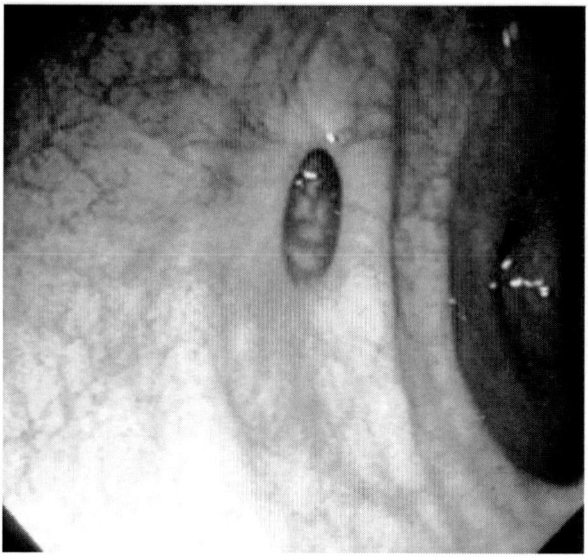

Figure 2. Diverticulum as seen on colonoscopy.

Computed Tomography

CT scan is the modality of choice in a patient of diverticular disease due to its high sensitivity and specificity. It not only establishes a diagnosis and rules out other differentials but also assesses the complications associated with diverticular disease. CT findings of localized bowel wall thickness >4 mm, increased soft tissue density and pericolic fat stranding and presence of diverticula suggests acute diverticulitis. In case of perforation, free air can be seen in peritoneal cavity. Abscess can be seen as a collection in area of inflammatory changes. The center of collection may contain air. Obstruction may be seen as dilated gut loops with air fluid levels in proximity to areas of inflammation. Extra-colonic air collection other than in the bowel suggests fistula. CT scan has the advantage of being noninvasive and there is no fear of increase in intraluminal pressure. It has an additional advantage of diagnosing extra luminal disorders such as ureteral obstruction and presence of distant abscess formation.

Magnetic Resonance Imaging (MRI)

It can be used as an alternative to ultrasonography, though generally not available in all the centers in emergency set up. These three- dimensional models may have a role in pre surgical planning with concurrent assessment of residual colon without any exposure to ionizing radiation. On MRI, features which are suggestive of acute diverticulitis include colonic wall thickening, presence of diverticula, peri-colonic exudates and edema. Although MRI avoids radiation, in most of the settings where CT and MRI is available, CT is utilized more expeditiously.

Trans Rectal Ultra Sonography (TRUS)

In selected cases of sigmoid diverticulitis it may be a useful adjuvant where facility for CT scan is not available.

Other Investigations

In patients with suspected or documented fistula formation, some other rele vant investigations may be utilized, which include cystoscopy, vaginoscopy, fistulogram and vaginogram.

Giant Colonic Diverticulum

Giant colonic diverticulum (GCD) was first described in French literature by Bonvin and Bonte in 1946. Since then, various names such as solitary air cyst, giant air cyst, colonic pneumocyst, encysted pneumatocele and giant diverticulum have been used for the same entity. These are poorly defined lesions without any clear definition and present as giant air filled cysts attached to colon. GCDs are rare clinical entities and most commonly present with pain abdomen. On examination, abdominal mass is the most common clinical finding. Although plain radiography may be enough for diagnosis, a CT can be done to delineate the anatomy. Surgical treatment is mandatory as they are associated with high complication rates. Diverticulectomy or segmental resection is the ideal surgical treatment with usually good results [37, 60].

TREATMENT

There has been an increasing trend in recent years to treat even patients having recurrent attacks of diverticulitis conservatively, although only in absence of any complications. That is why indications of surgery in an elective setting in absence of any complications are still controversial. Both laparoscopic and open surgical approaches have been performed to deal with such entities. Presently, various treatment modalities are being evaluated continuously in order to have the best possible therapeutic approach for this growing entity worldwide.

Management of the diverticulitis will be discussed briefly in this chapter as the same has been discussed in detail elsewhere in the book. Management of diverticulitis can be broadly discussed under following headings:

1) Acute uncomplicated diverticulitis, which can be further divided into:
    - Outpatient management
    - Inpatient management.

2) Acute complicated diverticulitis.

MANAGEMENT OF ACUTE UNCOMPLICATED DIVERTICULITIS

When diverticulitis is not associated with perforation, fistula, obstruction or abscess formation, it is known as uncomplicated diverticulitis and can be treated conservatively in most of the cases. Contrary to the previous teachings of resection after two attacks of uncomplicated and single attack of complicated diverticulitis, the recommendations of surgery are now individualized. A number of disease and patient related factors such as risk of subsequent attack, severity of recurrent attacks, risk of perforation or development of complications and risk of emergency surgery determine the management in the setting of uncomplicated diverticulitis.

Outpatient Management

Few patients with minor attacks of diverticulitis can be treated on outpatient basis with oral antibiotics and a clear liquid diet. Uncomplicated diverticulitis usually responds to the antibiotics and introduction of high fiber diet with marked improvement of symptoms in 48 hours. The antibiotics should target gram-negative rods and anaerobes. A broad spectrum antibiotic or a combination of metronidazole and ciprofloxacin should be used.

Inpatient Management

If the patient has severe pain and peritonitis is suspected, patient should be hospitalized and put on intravenous antibiotics and intravenous fluids. Analgesics and antispasmodics are added to improve patient comfort. Once the inflammation subsides, oral intake can be advised and before the patients are discharged, they should be advised a high fiber diet. Psyllium seed preparations should be prescribed to add bulk to the stool in order to minimize the segmentation. After the acute attack subsides, colonoscopic examination should be conducted at least 6 weeks later to rule out possibility of malignancy.

The risk of recurrence after an attack of diverticulitis has been quoted up to 30%, with individuals having a positive family history and CT finding of >5 cm of colonic segment of diverticulitis showing a higher rate of recurrence. A large number of studies have shown that the risk of complicated diverticulitis after an episode of uncomplicated diverticulitis is up to 5%. Sigmoidectomy is the choice of operation for the patients electively chosen for surgery after diverticulitis.

Management of Acute Complicated Diverticulitis

The complications of diverticulitis include abscess formation, obstruction, fistula, perforation and peritonitis. Complicated diverticulitis is associated with high rates of recurrent complications and high rates of mortality [61-63].

Abscess Formation

Diverticulitis in as many as 20% patients may be associated with **abscess** formation, mainly in the pelvis. The patient usually presents with pain, fever, leukocytosis and mass with tenderness may be elicited on per-abdominal, pelvic and rectal examination. The management usually depends upon the size of the abscess. An abscess <4 cm in size can be treated with antibiotics and analgesics whereas an abscess >4 cm in size usually needs a percutaneous or transanal drainage radiologically [41, 42, 43]. The patient is to be monitored for signs of improvement or deterioration. An elective surgery can be planned 6 weeks later after drainage of abscess wherein removal of the entire diseased, brittle colon should be performed [64, 65].

Fistula Formation

Colovesical fistula is most common complication, usually presenting with pneumaturia, faecaluria and polymicrobial urinary tract infection [44]. It is best diagnosed with a CT which shows air in the bladder in absence of history of prior instrumentation. It is necessary to exclude malignancy in such cases by colonoscopy, cystoscopy and cystogram. Fistula can be dealt with in a single stage with sigmoidectomy, pinching off fistula from bladder wall, closure of bladder wall, placement of omentum in between and catheterization with Foley's catheter [66, 67].

Colovaginal fistulas are almost exclusively present in women who have undergone hysterectomy for some reason. These patients present with passage of air and faeces through vagina and like in colovesical fistula, excluding malignancy is very important. Treatment should be followed on same lines like that for managing a colovesical fistula [67, 68].

Colocutaneous fistulas usually occur at the site of percutaneous drainage of abscess or result from anastomotic leak wherein inadequate resection of sigmoid colon is a major risk factor.

Obstruction

Stricture formation after diverticulitis is a major cause of obstruction. However the patients might not present with complete obstruction. As in other complications, exclusion of malignancy and other inflammatory conditions is mandatory. Strictures can be dealt with either stenting or simply by resection [68, 69, 70].

Perforation and Peritonitis

The perforated diverticulitis is one of the grave complication of diverticulitis and is classified according to the modified Hinchey classification as follows [60-63]:

- Stage 0- Mild clinical diverticulitis.
- Stage Ia- Pericolic inflammation/ phlegmon.
- Stage Ib- Pericolic abscess.
- Stage II- Pelvic, distant intra-abdominal or retroperitoneal abscess.
- Stage III- Generalized purulent peritonitis.
- Stage IV- Fecal peritonitis.

The management of perforation does not always necessitate need of emergent laparotomy. The objective findings of peritonitis and presence of toxicity is necessary for a patient to earn a laparotomy. The surgical options are diverse with much diverse advantages and disadvantages and depend upon the condition of the patient and intra operative findings and expertise of the surgeon. Surgical options include Hartmann's resection, sigmoid resection with primary anastomosis, and sigmoid resection with primary anastomosis with proximal diversion, on table lavage with primary anastomosis or laparoscopic lavage without resection [68-70]. Hartmann's procedure is the most common procedure performed for perforated diverticulitis with disadvantage of permanent stoma in about one thirds of patients. Fibrin glue with suture repair with omental patching has also been reported. However, emergency procedures have been associated with overall higher morbidity and mortality [71-74].

Principles of surgical management of diverticular disease suggest that Hartmann's procedure is a safe option in dealing with emergency surgical situations, however primary anastomosis can be taken into consideration in few. Elective resection is suggested for recurrent cases and definitive treatment of colo-vesical fistula might require resection procedure.

REFERENCES

[1] Bethesda, MD. (2001). *The Burden of Gastrointestinal Diseases*. American Gastroenterology Association.

[2] Papagrigoriadis, S., Debra S. and Koreli A. (2004). Impact of diverticular disease on hospital costs and activity. *Colorectal Dis*, 6: 81-84.

[3] Littre, A. 1700. Cited by: Finney JM. (1928). Diverticulitis and its surgical management. *Proc Interstate Post-Grad Med Assembly North Am*, 55: 57-65.

[4] Cruveilhier J. (1849). *Traite d' Anatomie Pathologique Generale* [*Treats of General Pathological Anatomy*], Vol.1. Paris, France: Bailliere.

[5] Graser, E.(1899). Das falsche Darmdivertikel [The wrong intestinal diverticulum]. *Arch Klin Chir*, 59: 638-647.

[6] Beer, E.(2000). Some pathological and clinical aspects of acquired diverticula of the intestine. *Colorectal Dis*, 7(1):107.

[7] Moynihan, B. (1907). The mimicry of malignant disease in large intestine. *Edinb Med J*, 1:1067.

[8] Case, JT. (1914).The roentgen demonstration of multiple diverticula of colon. *Am J Roentgenol*, 2: 654.

[9] E Quervain, F. (1914). Zur diagnose der erworbenen dickdarmdivertikel und der sigmoiditis diverticularis [For the diagnosis of acquired colon diverticula and sigmoiditis diverticularis]. *Dtsch Z Chir*, 128: 67.

[10] Hughes, LE. (1969).Postmortem survey of diverticular disease of the colon. Diverticulosis and diverticulitis. *Gut*, 10: 336-4.

[11] Kang, JY, Hoare, J. and Tinto, A.(2003).Diverticular disease of the colon on the rise: a study of hospital admissions in England between 1989/1990 and 1999/2000. *Aliment Pharmacol Ther*. 17:1189–95

[12] Painter, NS. and Burkitt, DP. (1975). Diverticular disease of colon: A 20th century problem. *Clinical Gastroenterology*, 4(1):3.

[13] Peery AF, Barrett PR, Park D et al. (2012 Feb) EPub 2011, Nov 4. A high fiber diet does not protect against asymptomatic diverticulosis. *Gastroenterol*, 142(2):266-72.

[14] Delvoux, M. (2003).Diverticular disease of colon in Europe: Epidemiology, impact on citizen health and prevention. *Aliment Pharmacol Ther*, 18 suppl. 3:71.

[15] Chan, CC., Lo KK., and Chung EC (1988). Colonic diverticulosis in Hong Kong: Distribution pattern and clinical significance. *Clinical Radiology*, 53(11): 842.

[16] Ngoi, SS, Chia, J. and Goh MY.(1992). Surgical management of Right colon diverticulitis. *Disease colon Rectum*, 35(8): 799.

[17] Markham, NI. and Li,AK.(1992). Diverticulitis of right colon. Experience from Hong Kong. *Gut*, 33(4): 547.

[18] Wang, FW, Chuang, HY. and Tu MS. (2015) E Pub 2015, April 11.Prevalence and risk factors of asymptomatic colorectal diverticulosis in Taiwan. *BMC Gastroenterol*, 15(1): 40.

[19] Wong, SK., Ho. YH., Leong, AP.and Seow -Choen F. (1997) Clinical behavior of complicated right-sided and left-sided diverticulosis. *Dis Colon Rectum*, 40: 344-348.

[20] Aldoori, WH., Giowannucci, EL. and Rimm EB. (1995). Prospective study of physical activity and risk of symptomatic diverticular disease in men. *Gut*, 36 (2): 276.

[21] Strait, LL., Liu, YL. and Aldoori WH. (2009) EPub 2008, Sep 25. Obesity increases the risk of diverticulitis and diverticular bleeding. *Gastroenterology*, 136(1): 115.

[22] Aldoori, WH., Giovannucci, EL. and Rimm EB. (1995). Prospective study of physical activity and the risk of symptomatic diverticular disease in men. *Gut*, 36(2):276–282. [PMC free article] [PubMed] [Google Scholar].

[23] Strate, LL., Liu, YL., Aldoori, WH., Syngal, S.and Giovannucci, EL. (2009). Obesity increases the risks of diverticulitis and diverticular bleeding. *Gastroenterology*, 136(1):115–122, e1. [PMC free article] [PubMed][Google Scholar].

[24] Jansen. A., Harenberg. S., Grenda,U. and Elsing C. (2009). Risk factors for colonic diverticular bleeding: a Westernized community based hospital study. *World J Gastroenterol*, 15(4):457–4 [PubMed] [Google Scholar].

[25] Yamada, A., Sugimoto, T. and Kondo S. (2008). Assessment of the risk factors for colonic diverticular hemorrhage. *Dis Colon Rectum*, 51(1):116–120. [PubMed] [Google Scholar].

[26] Aldoori, WH., Giovannucci, EL., Rimm, EB., Wing, AL., Trichopoulos, DV.and Willett WC. (1995). A prospective study of alcohol, smoking, caffeine, and the risk of symptomatic diverticular disease in men. *Ann Epidemiol*, 5(3):221228. [PubMed] .

[27] Hjern, F., Wolk, A. and Hakansson, N. (2011 July). Smoking and risk of diverticular disease in women. *BRJ Surgery* 98(7): 997-1002. E Pub. 2011, April 4.

[28] Humes, DJ., Fleming, KM. and Spiller, RC (2011 Feb). Concurrent drug use and risk of perforated colonic diverticular disease: A population based case control study. *Gut*, 60(2): 2019-24. E Pub 2010, Oct 12.

[29] Strait, LL., Liu, YL. and Huang ES . (2011). Use of aspirin or NSAIDs increases risk of diverticulitis and diverticular bleeding. *Gastroenterology*, 140:1427.

[30] Aldoori, WH., Giowannucci, EL. and Rimm EB. (1998). Use of acetaminophen and NSAIDs: A prospective study and risk of symptomatic diverticular disease in men. *Arch Fam Med*, 7: 255.

[31] Morris, CR., Harvey, IM. and Stebbings WS. (2003). Do calcium channel blockers and anti muscarinics protect against perforated colonic diverticular disease? A case control study. *Gut*, 52: 1737.

[32] Majurie, LH., Song, m., and Strate LE . (2013).Higher serum level of Vitamin D associated with reduced risk of diverticulitis. *Clinical Gastroenterol Hepatol*, 11: 1631.

[33] Comparato, G., Pilotto, A., Franzè, A., Franceschi, M. and Di Mario F. (2007).Diverticular disease in the elderly. *Dig Dis*, 25(2):151–159. [PubMed] [Google Scholar].

[34] Trivedi CD, Das KM, NDSG.(2008). Emerging therapies for diverticular disease of the colon. *J Clin Gastroenterol*, 42(10):1145–1151. [PubMed] [Google Scholar].

[35] Leung, DYM., Glagov, S., Mathews, MB. (1976). Cyclic stretching stimulates synthesis of matrix components of arterial smooth muscle cells in vivo. *Science*, 191: 475-477.

[36] Sheth, A.and Floch, M.(2009) Probiotics and diverticular disease. *Nutr Clin Pra*, 24(1):41–44. [PubMed] [Google Scholar].

[37] Tursi A, Brandimarte G, Giorgetti G M, Elisei W.(2006). Mesalazine and/or Lactobacillus casei in preventing recurrence of symptomatic uncomplicated diverticular disease of the colon: a prospective, randomized, open-label study. *J Clin Gastroenterol*, 40(4):312–316. [PubMed] [Google Scholar].

[38] Tursi, A., Brandimarte, G., Giorgetti, GM., Elisei, W. and Aiello F. (2007).Balsalazide and /or high-potency probiotic mixture (VSL#3) in maintaining remission after attack of acute, uncomplicated diverticulitis of the colon. *Int J Colorectal Dis*, 22(9):1103–1108. [PubMed] [Google Scholar].

[39] Arfwidsson, S., Kock, N., Lehmann, L. and Winberg T. (1964) Pathogenesis of multiple diverticula of the sigmoid colon in diverticular diseases. *Acta Chir Scand*,; 342(Suppl):1–68. [PubMed] [Google Scholar].

[40] Parks, TG. and Connell, AM. (1969). Motility studies in diverticular disease of the colon. *Gut*, 10(7):534–542. [PMC free article] [PubMed] [Google Scholar]

[41] Snape, WJ. Jr., Carlson, GM. and Cohen, S. (1976). Colonic myoelectric activity in the irritable bowel syndrome. *Gastroenterology*,70(3):326–330. [PubMed] [Google Scholar].

[42] Taylor, I., and Duthie, HL.(1976). Bran tablets and diverticular disease. *BMJ*, 1(6016):988–990. [PMC free article] [PubMed] [Google Scholar].

[43] Bassotti G, Battaglia E, Spinozzi F, Pelli MA, Tonini M. (2001). Twenty-four hour recordings of colonic motility in patients with diverticular disease: evidence for abnormal motility and propulsive

activity. *Dis Colon Rectum*, 44 (12):1814–1820. [PubMed] [Google Scholar].

[44] Tomita, R., Fujisaki, S., Tanjoh, K. and Fukuzawa M. (2000). Role of nitric oxide in the left-sided colon of patients with diverticular disease. *Hepato-gastroenterology*, 47(33):692–696. [PubMed] [Google Scholar].

[45] Milner P, Crowe R, Kamm MA, Lennard-Jones JE, Burnstock G. (1990).Vasoactive intestinal polypeptide levels in sigmoid colon in idiopathic constipation and diverticular disease. *Gastroenterology*, 993):666–675. [PubMed] [Google Scholar].

[46] Costedio, MM., Coates,MD. and Danielson AB. (2008). Serotonin signaling in diverticular disease. *J Gastrointest Surg*, 12(8):1439–1445. [PMC free article] [PubMed] [Google Scholar].

[47] Hodgson, J. (1972). Effect of methylcellulose on rectal and colonic pressures in treatment of diverticular disease. *BMJ*, 3(5829):729–731. [PMC free article] [PubMed] [Google Scholar

[48] Painter NS, Truelove SC, Ardran GM, Tuckey M.(1968). Segmentation and the localization of intraluminal pressure in the human colon, with special reference to the pathogenesis of colonic diverticula. *Gastroenterology*, 54 (Suppl 4):778–780. [PubMed] [Google Scholar].

[49] Painter, NS. (1964).The aetiology of diverticulosis of the colon with special reference to the action of certain drugs on the behaviour of the colon. *Ann R Coll Surg Engl*, 34:98–119. [PMC free article] [PubMed] [Google Scholar].

[50] West, AB. (2006).The pathology of diverticulosis: classical concepts and mucosal changes in diverticula. *J Clin Gastroenterol*, 40 (Suppl 3):S126–S131. [PubMed] [Google Scholar].

[51] Stump, M., Cao, W. and Klinge U. (2001).Increased distribution of collagen type III and reduced expression of matrix metalloproteinase1 in patients with diverticular disease. *Int J Colorectal Dis*, 16: 271-275.

[52] Chappius, CW.and Cohn I Jr. Acute colonic diverticulitis. (1988). *Surg Clin North Am*, 68:301–312. [PubMed] [Google Scholar].

[53] Farmakis N., Tudor, RG. and Keighley MR. (1994).The 5-year natural history of complicated diverticular disease. *Br J Surg*, 81: 733–735. [PubMed] [Google Scholar].

[54] Boles, RS Jr., Jordan SM. (1958).The clinical significance of diverticulosis. *Gastroenterology*, 35:579. [PubMed] [Google Scholar].

[55] Parks, TG. (1969).Natural history of diverticular disease of the colon. A review of 521 cases. *BMJ*, 639–642. [PMC free article] [PubMed] [Google Scholar].

[56] Schoetz DJ. (1999).Diverticular disease of the colon: a century old problem. *Dis Colon Rectum*, 42: 703–709. [PubMed] [Google Scholar].

[57] Anthony, l.I. (1997). Diverticular disease of the colon. In: Sebeston DC, Lyerly HK, *text book of surgery, the biological basis of modern surgical practice*, 15th edition W.B. Saunders company, 982-993.

[58] Letwin, ER. (1982). Diverticulitis of the colon: Clinical review of acute presentation and management. *Am. J. surg*., 143:579.

[59] Choong, CK. and Frizelle, FA. (1998).Giant colonic diverticulum: report of four cases and review of the literature. *Dis Colon Rectum*, 41:1178-1186.

[60] Champman, J., Davies, M. and Wolff B. (2005). Complicated diverticulitis. Is it time to rethink the rules? *Ann Surg*, 242(31): 576-583.

[61] Farmakis, N., Tudor, RG. and Keighley, MR.(1997). The 5 year natural history of complicated diverticular disease. *Br J Surg*, 81(32):733-735.

[62] Norman, SW., O'connell, PR. and WM, Andrew. (2018). In *Bailey and Love's Short Practice of Surgery*, 27th Edition vol. 2(33); 1276.

[63] Hackford, AW. and Schoetz DJ. (1985). Surgical management of complicated diverticulitis: the Lahey Clinic experience, 1967 to 1982. *Dis Colon Rectum*, 28:317–321. [PubMed] [Google Scholar].

[64] Wedell, J. and Banzhaf, G. (1997). Surgical management of complicated colonic diverticulitis. *Br J Surg*, 84: 380–383. [PubMed] [Google Scholar].

[65] Lambert, ME. and Knox, RA. (1986). Management of the septic complications of diverticular disease. *Br J Surg*, 73: 576–579. [PubMed] [Google Scholar] 4.

[66] Kirsch, GM., Hampel, N., Shuck, JM, and Resnick, MI. (1991) Diagnosis and management of vesico-enteric fistulas. *Surg. gyneco*, Obstet, 173:91.

[67] Woods, RJ., Lavery, IC., Fazio, VW., jagelman, DG., and weakley FL. (1988).Internal fistulas in diverticular disease. *Dis. colon rectum*, 31:591.

[68] Kronborg O. (1993).Treatment of perforated sigmoid diverticulitis: a prospective randomized trial. *Br J Surg*, 80:505–507. [PubMed] [Google Scholar].

[69] Griffen, WO Jr. (1976).Management of the acute complications of diverticular disease: acute perforation of colonic diverticula. *Dis Colon Rectum*, 19:293–295. [PubMed] [Google Scholar].

[70] Hinchey, EJ., Schaal, PG. and Richards, GK. (1978). Treatment of perforated diverticular disease of the colon. *Adv surg*, 12:85-109.

[71] Eng, K., Ranson, JHC, and Locolia, SA. (1977). Resection of the perforated segment. A significant advance in treatment of diverticulitis with free perforation or abscess. *Am. J. Surg*, 133:67.

[72] Labs, JD., Sarr, MG., Fishman, EK., Siegelman, SS. and Cameron, JL. (1988). Complications of acute diverticulitis of colon: Improved early diagnosis with computerised tomography. *Am J surg*, 155: 331.

[73] Haglund U., Hellberg R., Johnsen C., and Hulte L. (1977). Complicated diverticular disease of the sigmoid colon. An analysis of short and long term outcome in 392 patients. *Ann. Chir. Gynaecol*, 68: 41.

[74] Makela, J., Kiviniemi, H. and laitinen S. (2002). Prevelance of perforated sigmoid diverticulitis is increasing. *Dis Colon Rectum*, 45:955-961.

In: Diverticulitis: Diagnosis and Treatment ISBN: 978-1-53618-081-7
Editors: Shams-ul-Bari et al.

Chapter 2

RADIOLOGY OF DIVERTICULITIS

M. Farooq Mir*
DNB Radiodiagnosis, Department of radiodiagnosis Skims,
Medical College Srinagar, Jammu and Kashmir, India

ABSTRACT

Various radiologic investigations have been used for the evaluation of patients suspected of having complicated diverticular disease. Each has its own advantages and limitations. USG has been widely used, but its operator dependency and subjective interpretation has limited its use. Computed Tomography has been proved by many studies to have the highest accuracy in detection of diverticulitis. It is also the most valuable investigation to rule out other disorders with similar presentation. CT scan is valuable in defining the location and extent of the inflammatory process, thereby allowing appropriate clinical management. In view of the obvious advantages, CT scan is considered as the initial radiologic imaging test of choice in the United States.

Although, MRI has demonstrated similar or better sensitivity and specificity as compared to CT scan in several early studies of patients and may eventually supplement CT, but its high cost and current limited availability does not make it currently feasible for routine use.

* Corresponding Author's Email: mirfarooq_99@yahoo.com.

INTRODUCTION

Colonic diverticulosis (plural diverticuloses) refers to the presence of multiple diverticula. Diverticula are small sacs of mucosa and submucosa (Figure 1) that protrude through the muscle layer of the wall of the intestinal loop, between the taenia coli and the mesentery, at the point of penetration of the blood vessel [1]. It is quite distinct from diverticulitis which describes inflammation and infection of one or multiple diverticula [2]. Medical and surgical therapy for diverticulosis is initiated primarily for the complications of diverticulitis and lower gastrointestinal haemorrhage from a diverticular source.

Diverticulosis of the colon continues to rise in prevalence, especially in Western countries, where up to two-thirds of the population older than 70 years of age are estimated to have the disorder [3]. The incidence of diverticulosis increases from 5% at the of 40 years to 30% at the age of 60 years and 50-80% by the age of 80 [4]. Colonic diverticula are most common in the sigmoid colon and, to a lesser extent, in the descending colon. Although usually the entire colon can be affected, however 15% patients have right-sided diverticula only. In patients from Asia, right-sided diverticula are more common, and can either be single or multiple. The entity of giant colonic diverticulum is uncommon and usually arises from the sigmoid colon [5].

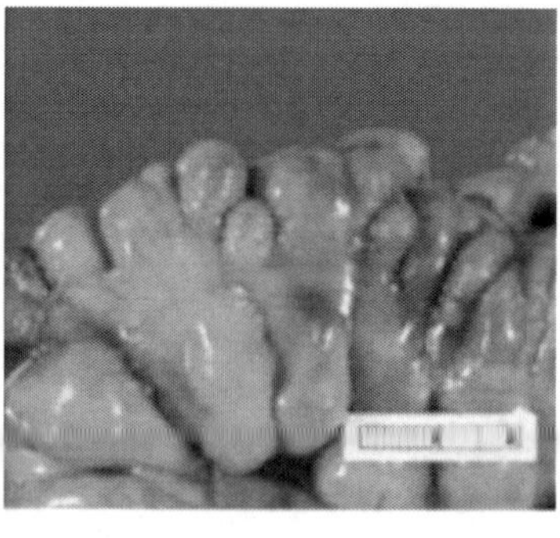

Figure 1. Multiple Diverticuli in colon.

RADIOLOGY

Diverticula range in size from a few millimetres to a few centimetres [6]. Objective confirmation of the extent of the disease process by radiologic examination has been motivated over the last three decades because of inaccuracies in diagnosis and management. Plain radiographs, endoscopy, contrast enema, ultrasound (US) and computed tomography (CT) have all been studied as adjuncts to the diagnosis of complicated diverticular disease [7]. Recently, studies on the application of MRI in diverticular disease have also been reported [8].

PLAIN RADIOGRAPHY

The initial study for all patients who present to the emergency department with abdominal pain possibly due to diverticulitis is an abdominal X-rays. Many of the abnormalities on x-ray are nonspecific. However in some patients we may find an abnormal finding such as ileus or obstructive gas pattern, a soft tissue mass, or Pneumo-peritoneum. Free air may be present in up to 12% of cases. While the plain films may suggest a diagnosis of diverticulitis, other studies are required for confirmation prior to the initiation of medical or surgical therapy [9]. Plain film radiography however may fail to demonstrate the small contained perforations and is not sensitive for other complications such as abscess and fistula [10].

CONTRAST ENEMA

Until the 1980s when it was replaced by CT, contrast enema was the primary imaging modality for colonic diverticulitis. Today, barium enema is not performed. When performed for presumed acute diverticulitis, a water-soluble contrast enema (CE) is used. In the appropriate clinical setting, contrast enema findings of fold thickening, segmental spasm, sinus tract, fistula, mass effect from abscess and extra luminal free or contained contrast may be demonstrated and can be diagnostic of acute diverticulitis. Both single and double contrast barium enemas are able to demonstrate diverticula as barium-filled out-pouchings (Figure 2 and Figure 3). When seen 'en face' they can look similar to polyps but can be distinguished by the presence of contrast pooling within the diverticulum and forming a meniscus. Even if seen on a recumbent overhead film, the two can usually be separated. Contrast enemas are most useful in the setting of chronic diverticulitis for follow-up of patients when diverticulitis is suspected. Contrast enema is a more time-consuming investigation for the patients when compared with other imaging modalities like CT, and generally it is not a good test to rule out other disorders with similar presentation [11]. Contrast enema is not as sensitive as CT (80 to 92% for CE versus up to 99% for CT) [12]. The absence of apparent diverticulosis requires reassessment of the diagnosis. The most reliable radiologic sign of diverticulitis seen on contrast enema examination is the appearance of extra luminal contrast [13]. Contrast may track through a perforated diverticulum into a sinus tract or abscess cavity or may connect with an adjacent organ as a fistula. Colo-venous and colo-salpingeal fistulae demonstrated with barium contrast have been reported [14]. While contrast enema remains an important modality in the diagnosis and evaluation of colonic neoplasms and inflammatory diseases, its utility in evaluating patients with acute diverticulitis is diminishing. Over the past 30 years its disadvantages and inferiority to newer modalities such as USG abdomen and CT abdomen have been demonstrated.

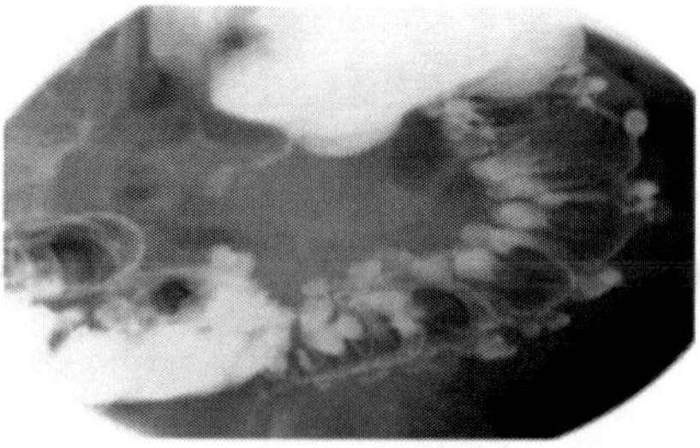

Figure 2. Double contrast barium study showing multiple Diverticuli.

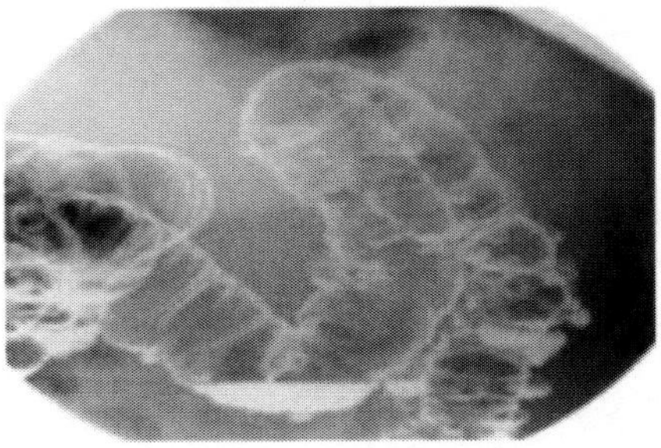

Figure 3. Barium contrast study showing multiple Diverticuli.

ULTRASONOGRAPHY

High-resolution real-time sonography, although not commonly used in the United States for this purpose, has been proven to have an effective role in diagnosing acute diverticulitis and its complications [15]. The use of USG for imaging in appendicitis and inflammatory bowel disease preceded its use in diverticular disease and laid the foundation for a greater knowledge of echographic appearances of normal and abnormal bowel [16]. The normal colonic wall measures 3 mm or less in thickness and can seldom be recognized on routine ultasonography. Accurate examination of the sigmoid colon relies on differentiating the colonic lumen from that of the small bowel. This difference can be ascertained by the typical location of the sigmoid colon, its lack of valvulae conniventes, and absence of typical small bowel peristalsis. Fleischer and associates were the first to conclude that a bowel wall greater than 5 mm in thickness should be considered pathologic [17]. Sonographic examination in patients with acute diverticulitis demonstrates hypoechoic thickening of the wall of the involved segment of colon greater than 5 mm with a central echogenic focus. In the transverse orientation, this finding results into a "target" or "pseudokidney" appearance, as described by Parulekar. In longitudinal sectioning, a more tubular pattern with narrowing or complete obstruction of the lumen is seen. Repeat examination during a resolving episode of acute diverticulitis will demonstrate regression of the colonic thickening. A rigid zone of increased echogenicity adjacent to the colon wall represents omental or pericolic fat encasing the inflammatory process. Intramural and extramural diverticula can also be visualized as hyperechoic foci within the inflamed wall of the colon. These foci represent air or residue within the lumen of the diverticulum causing some associated acoustic shadowing [18]. Diverticular abscesses can present with a spectrum of ultrasonic findings but usually appear as predominantly cystic masses containing echogenic debris. Occasionally they have the appearance of solid lesions, or they may contain gas. Abscesses are differentiated from free peritoneal fluid by their resistance to change, shape, or location under external compression. Thickening of adjacent bowel loops secondary to edema and inflammation and a surrounding rigid zone of increased echogenicity are exhibited by almost all intra abdominal abscesses. Intramural abscesses appear as well circumscribed anechoic masses within a thickened colonic wall. Infrequently, sinus tracts connecting abscesses with the colonic wall are also visible [19]. Abdominal USG is often limited by overlying gas that obscures the diseased segment and may produce false negative results. This problem is accentuated by obesity as well as acute diverticulitis where inflammation may cause a localized ileus in neighbouring small bowel segments. Disease in the distal sigmoid colon is also more difficult to assess, as it can be poorly accessible to the USG due to interference from the bladder and other pelvic structures. Recently, some institutions have employed transrectal sonography with an end-firing endocavitary probe to complement trans-abdominal sonography [20].

Findings of Acute Diverticulitis on Ultrasound Evaluation

- Colonic wall >5 mm
- "Target"/"pseudokidney"sign
- Diverticulum
- Pain/tenderness on compression of involved area
- Diverticular abscess (cystic masses)
- Intramural abscesses
- Colovesical fistula.

COMPUTED TOMOGRAPHY

Computed tomography (CT) is considered as the method of choice in the protocols established by the American Society of Colon and Rectal Surgeons in Colonic Diverticulosis and Diverticulitis, because it allows rapid diagnosis and has an accuracy of over 90% [21]. The optimal management of diverticulitis requires a complete appraisal of peritoneal involvement, including the location and extent of inflammation, and the presence or absence of complications. CT enables accurate assessment of both the intraluminal and extra-luminal components of the disease as well as involvement of other nearby organs and distant disease. CT is also invaluable in deciding operative versus non-operative therapy and response to medical therapy [22]. Lieberman and Haaga first documented the CT features of acute diverticulitis as bowel wall thickening, increased soft tissue density within the pericolic fat secondary to inflammation, and soft tissue masses representing either phlegmon or abscess [23]. Both conventional and helical techniques have been used for diverticular disease. Optimal scanning requires oral, intravenous, and rectal contrast. Many emergent abdominal and pelvic CT scans are performed, however, with only oral and intravenous contrast. CT with intravenous and oral contrast administration alone is reported to be 93% sensitive and 100% specific [24]. CT with colonic contrast introduced retrograde without oral or intravenous contrast has produced sensitivities between 93% and 97% with 100% specificity. When Rao and colleagues studied the use of helical CT with only colonic contrast, they found that in addition to its high sensitivity (93%), the technique could be performed immediately without the additional risks of intravenous contrast and discomfort of contrast administered orally [25]. On CT images, the normal colon appears to have a thin wall with haustrations and no apparent diverticula. In contrast, segmental thickening of the colonic wall, defined as a thickness of more than 4 mm on a scan perpendicular to or through the long axis of a slightly distended colon lumen, is a common finding in diverticulitis [26]. Fine linear stranding within the pericolic inflammatory process is also often present. Diverticula are identified as flask-shaped structures filled with air, barium, or faecal material seen in cross-section projecting through the wall of the colon (Figure 4).

The presence of diverticula in the involved segment is helpful in distinguishing diverticulitis from other inflammatory conditions that affect the sigmoid colon, such as inflammatory bowel disease and ischemia (27). The arrow-head sign is seen as a contrast material collecting in an arrow-head shape adjacent to the focally inflamed colonic wall. An inflamed diverticulum is recognized as a rounded, paracolic out pouching centered within an area of pericolonic inflammation. It has similar attenuation to soft tissue, calcium, barium, or air. The arrow-head sign and the finding of an inflamed diverticulum have sensitivity rates of 27% and 33%, respectively. Significantly, the specificity of these CT findings is 100% and, when present, they aid in the definitive diagnosis of diverticulitis and the exclusion of other colonic inflammatory processes (28). Thickening of the root of the sigmoid mesocolon appears as a high-attenuation line along the pelvic wall anterior to the iliopsoas muscle. Often a thin rim of fluid may track along this region and is a sensitive finding for acute diverticulitis. Mesenteric venous engorgement is also commonly noted [29]. Micro perforation of a diverticulum often leads to the development of focal contained collections appearing as small extra luminal pockets of air, gas bubbles, or extravasation of rectal contrast material. This situation may still be amenable to medical management. On the other hand, extra luminal air identified on CT scan in the mesenteric venous branches and portal venous branches is a rare but ominous finding of sigmoid diverticulitis, requiring urgent surgical intervention [30].

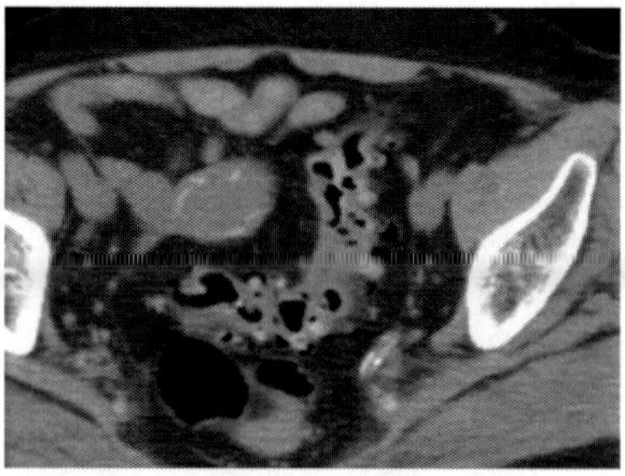

Figure 4. CT showing multiple Diverticuli in colon.

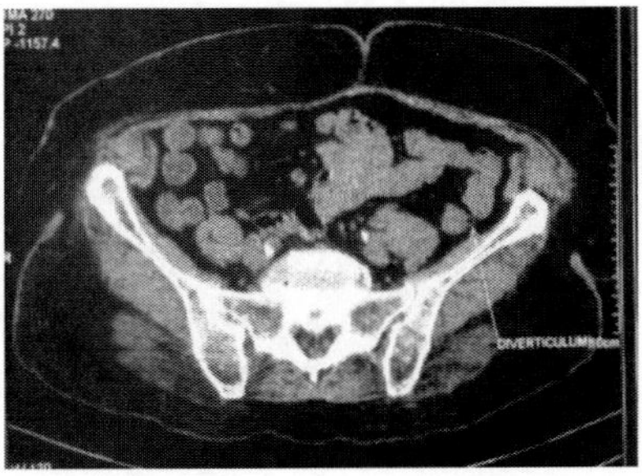

Figure 5. CT showing Colonic Diverticulum (axial view).

Complications are present in up to 30% of cases of diverticulitis and usually necessitate radiological or surgical intervention. The most common is a peridiverticular abscess followed by colovesical, colovaginal, or colocutaneous fistulae. Abscesses are usually peri-colonic or intramural and appear as an abnormal fluid collection within an area of inflammatory changes. The centre of the collection may contain air, air-fluid levels, or tissue with low attenuation representing necrotic debris. Distant abscesses in the flank, psoas muscle, subphrenic space, and liver can also occur from both hematogenous spread and distant intraperitoneal seeding of ruptured diverticula [31].

Findings of Acute Diverticulitis on Computed Tomography in Decreasing Frequency of Occurrence
Pericolic inflammation/edema
Diverticula Colonic wall thickening (>4 mm)
Pericolic abscess
Arrowhead sign
Inflamed diverticulum
Fistula
Extra pelvic abscess
Colonic obstruction
Intramural sinus tracks
Small bowel obstruction
Ureteral obstruction

MAGNETIC RESONANCE IMAGING

The possible role of magnetic resonance imaging (MRI) in inflammatory conditions of the gastrointestinal tract has only recently been evaluated. MRI does not require the intravenous, oral, and rectal contrast necessary for optimal CT scans. In addition, MRI is not limited by poor visualization due to overlying gas and fat and by the requirement for experienced radiologists and technicians that has limited the use of US in this country. The specific MR imaging diagnosis of acute diverticulitis is based on the findings of at least one diverticulum, pericolic exudation and edema, and thickening of the colonic wall. In addition, segmental narrowing and ascites are considered supportive of the diagnosis of diverticulitis [4]. Abscesses, perforations and other complications of diverticular disease have not yet been critically assessed by using MRI. However, one would expect that the use of intravenous contrast media with acquisition of high-resolution T1-weighted images should allow clear delineation of these complications with accuracy equal or superior to CT and US (17). Despite the reported accuracy of MRI in several small series of patients, we do not endorse its widespread use because its relative advantages appear outweighed by higher cost, limited availability, and contraindication with patients having metallic implants [8].

NUCLEAR IMAGING

Nuclear imaging has limited use in the diagnostic evaluation of diverticulitis and is primarily used to localize septic foci not found with other imaging modalities. Radio-pharmaceuticals, using Indium-labelled white blood cells and Gallium citrate are the two current options available. Neither agent is able to differentiate between an abscess and an inflammatory phlegmon (10).

Conclusion

Various radiologic modalities exist for the evaluation of patients suspected of having complicated diverticular disease. Each has its own advantages and limitations. USG has a proven track record in European countries, but its operator variability and subjective interpretation have limited its use in the United States. As shown in multiple studies, CT consistently has the highest accuracy in detection of diverticulitis. It is also the most capable modality for diagnosing alternative conditions. CT scans permit the complete evaluation of the location and extent of the inflammatory process, allowing appropriate clinical management. Furthermore, it can aid in the non-operative treatment of complicated diverticulitis by allowing percutaneous drainage of abscesses and permitting interval surgery without the need for a colostomy. Asa result, CT scanning continues to be the initial radiologic imaging test of choice in the United States. MRI has demonstrated similar or better sensitivities and specificities to CT scanning in small studies of patients and may eventually supplant CT. Its high cost and current limited availability do not make it feasible for routine use at this time. Further studies comparing it to CT scan in larger groups of patients are needed to determine its future role in the management of diverticular diseases.

References

[1] Tiferes, D.A., Jayanthi, S. K., Liguori, A. A.(2011). L. Cólon. reto e apêndice. In: D'Ippolito G., Caldana R. P., editores. *Gastrointestinal. Série CBR* [*CBR Series*]. 1ª ed. Rio de Janeiro: Editora Sarvier, P. no. 203-52.

[2] Avunduk C.(2008). Diagnosis and therapy. In Lippincott Williams & Wilkins. *Manual of Gastroenterology*, ISBN: 0781769744.

[3] Parks T. G.(1975). Natural history of diverticular disease of the colon. *Clin Gastroenterol*, 4:53-69.

[4] McPhee, S. J., Tierney, L. M. and Papadakis M. A.(2007). *Current medical diagnosis and treatment.* McGraw-Hill Professional. ISBN: 0071472479.

[5] Doherty G. M. and Way L. W.(2006). *Current surgical diagnosis & treatment*. McGraw-Hill Medical, ISBN: 007142315X.

[6] Horton, K. M., Corl, F. M. and Fishman E. K.(2000). CT evaluation of the colon: inflammatory disease. *Radiographics,* 20 (2): 399-418.

[7] Freeman S. R. and McNally P. R. (1993) Diverticulitis. *Med Clin North Am* 77: 1149-1167.

[8] Heverhagen, J. T., Zielke, A., Ishaque, N., Bohrer, T., El-Sheik, M., and Klose K. J.(2001). Acute colonic diverticulitis: visualization in magnetic resonance imaging. *Magnetic Resonance Imaging*,19:1275-1277.

[9] Field, S., Guy, P. J. and Upsdell, S. M..(1985). The erect abdominal radiograph in the acute abdomen: should its routine use be abandoned? *BMJ*, 290:1934-1936.

[10] Destigter K. K. and Keating D. P.(2009). Imaging update: acute colonic diverticulitis; *Clinics in colon and rectal surgery,* vol 22 (3); 147-155.

[11] Hulnick, D. H., Megibow, A. J., Balthazar, E. J., Gordon, R. B., Surapenini, R. and Bosniak M. A.(1987). Perforated colorectal neoplasms: correlation of clinical, contrast enema, and CT examinations. *Radiology* 164(3):611-615.

[12] Baker, M. E. (2008). Imaging and interventional techniques in acute left-sided diverticulitis. *J Gastrointest Surg*, 12(8):1314-1317.

[13] Chappuis, C. W. and Cohn, I. Jr. (1988). Acute colonic diverticulitis. *Surg Clin North Am,* 68:301-313.

[14] Williams, S. M. and Nolan, D. J.(1999). Colo-salpingeal fistula: a rare complication of colonic diverticular disease. *Eur Radiol* 9:1432-1433.

[15] Parulekar, S. G.(1985). Sonography of colonic diverticulitis. *J Ultrasound Med,* 4:659-666.

[16] Pozniak, M., Scanlan, K. and Yandow, D.(1987). Ultrasound in the evaluation of bowel disorders. *Sem Ultrasound CT MR*, 8:366-384.

[17] Incesu L., Coskun A., Selcuk M. B., Akan H., Sozubir S., Bernay F. Acute appendicitis: MR imaging and Sonographic correlation. *Am J Roentgenol* 1997; 168:669-674.

[18] Schwerk, W. B., Schwarz, S. and Rothmund, M.(1992). Sonography in acute colonic diverticulitis. A prospective study. *Dis Colon Rectum*, 35:1077-1084.

[19] Verbanck, J., Lambrecht, S. and Rutgeerts L.(1989) Can sonography diagnose acute colonic diverticulitis in patients with acute intestinal inflammation? A prospective study. *J Clin Ultra- sound*, 17:661-666.

[20] Hollerweger, A., Rettenbacher, T., Macheiner, P., Brunner, W., and Gritzmann N. Sigmoid diverticulitis: value of transrectal sonography in addition to transabdominal sonography. *AJR Am J Roentgenol* 2000; 175:1155-1160.

[21] Andeweg, C. S., Mulder, I. M., and Felt-Bersma, R. J. (2013). Guidelines of diagnostics and treatment of acute left-sided colonic diverticulitis. *Dig Surg*. 30:278-92.

[22] Gore, R. M. and Goldberg, H. I.(1982). Computed tomographic evaluation of the gastrointestinal tract in diseases other than first-degree adenocarcinoma. *Radiol Clin North Am*. 20:781-796.

[23] Birnbaum B. A.and Balthazar E. J.(1994). CT of appendicitis and diverticulitis. *Radiol. Clin North Am*, 32:885-898.

[24] Cho, K. C., Morehouse, H. T., Alteman, D. D. and Thornhill B. A.(1990) Sigmoid diverticulitis: diagnostic role of CT comparison with barium enema studies. *Radiology* 176:111-115.

[25] Rao, P. M., Rhea, J. T. and Novelline R. A. (1998). Helical CT with only colonic contrast material for diagnosing diverticulitis: prospective evaluation of 150 patients. *AJR Am J Roentgenol* 170:1445-1449.

[26] Ambrosetti, P., Jenny, A., Becker, C., Terrier, F. and Morel, P.(2000). Acute left colonic diverticulitis-compared performance of computed tomography and water-soluble contrast enema. *Dis Colon Rectum*, 43:1363-1367.

[27] Lieberman, J. M. and Haaga, J. R.(1983). Computed tomography of diverticulitis. *J Comput Assist Tomography*, 7:431-433.

[28] Rao, P. M. and Rhea, J. T.(1998). Colonic diverticulitis: evaluation of the arrowhead sign and the inflamed diverticulum for CT diagnosis. *Radiology,* 209: 775-779.
[29] Balthazar, E.(1994). Diverticular disease. In *Textbook of Gastrointestinal Radiology.* Philadelphia, PA: Saunders; 1072-1097.
[30] Molitch, H. I. (1996). Septic thrombophlebitis of the inferior mesenteric vein complicating sigmoid diverticulitis: CT findings. *AJR Am J Roentgenol,* 167:1014-1016.
[31] White, T. B., Allen, H. A. and III, Ives C. E.(1998). Portal and mesenteric vein gas in diverticulitis: CT findings. *AJR Am J Roentgenol,* 171:525-526.

In: Diverticulitis: Diagnosis and Treatment ISBN: 978-1-53618-081-7
Editors: Shams-ul-Bari et al.

Chapter 3

NON-ANTIBIOTIC TREATMENT OF UNCOMPLICATED ACUTE DIVERTICULITIS

Javier Serrano González[1,*],
Laura Román García de León[2]
and Jesús Gabriel García Schiever[3]
[1]GI Surgery, Hospital Universitario de Torrejón, Madrid, Spain
[2]GI Surgery, Hospital Universitario Puerta de Hierro Majadahonda, Madrid, Spain
[3]GI Surgery, Hospital General Universitario de Ciudad Real, Ciudad Real, Spain

ABSTRACT

Treatment of acute diverticulitis includes rest to the digestive tract, analgesia and broad spectrum antibiotics. This can be carried out as an outpatient treatment along with a regular follow up. However, there are studies conducted during last few years which have proved that non-antibiotic treatment could be safe in selected patients. The benefits of this therapeutic approach are based on eluding the adverse effects of any

* Corresponding Author's Email: javierserranogdr@gmail.com.

antibiotic based treatment, such as allergic reactions, development of drug resistance or other infectious effects.

In order to explain this different strategy, we have to consider that there is not a proven physiopathological theory for this disease. For decades, the most accepted theory has been that the acute diverticulitis originates as diverticular micro-perforations associated with bacterial translocation in every case. In the past few years, some theories suggest an inflammatory cause or a local immunological alteration as the origin of non-complicated acute diverticulitis. If no systemic response is involved, perhaps antibiotics could be avoided.

The non-antibiotic treatment comprises of partial rest to the digestive tract along with analgesic and anti-inflammatory drugs. The patient is discharged from the emergency ward with a clear liquid diet for the first 48 hours, followed by a low-fiber diet. At the same time, the patient is treated with an alternate regime of analgesics (acetaminophen) and NSAIDs.

Since these patients are treated as outpatients, a proper follow-up is mandatory, preferably by a colo-proctologist. This specialist will decide if control imaging is necessary or, although more infrequent nowadays, even a colonoscopy.

INTRODUCTION

Complications related with diverticular disease are one of the main gastrointestinal reasons for admission at the Emergency Ward. Its prevalence has been increasing in the past decades. At present it is considered that at 40 years of age, 20% of the population is suffering from this disease. This percentage is as high as 60% at 60 years and 75% in the population over 80 years. It has been classically accepted that clinical manifestations of diverticular disease appear in 10-25% of cases, but recent studies indicate an incidence of symptoms of 1-4% [1] and a recurrence rate of 15-30% [2]. These complications account for approximately 300,000 hospital admissions, 1.5 million inpatient care days and a direct cost of 2.4 billion dollars annually in the United States [3].

With this data in mind, an increasingly conservative approach, developed recently in the management of this disease, has been gaining importance and has been found to be a safe option for patients with uncomplicated acute diverticulitis. Surgical treatment is now restricted to severe cases of acute diverticulitis or in recurrent and chronic cases with significant loss of quality of life. This aggressive course of action has to be personalized in each case, and its morbidity and mortality have to be always taken into account.

This chapter is going to address a suggested treatment for non-complicated forms of diverticular disease, apart from the usual management using broad spectrum antibiotics in today's practice.

Uncomplicated acute diverticulitis (UAD) is defined as the clinical condition characterized by low abdominal pain (more frequently in the left iliac fossa or hypogastrium), associated with diverticular inflammation with or without affecting mesenteric fat, diagnosed with radiologic imaging [4]. It excludes cases with bowel obstruction, hemorrhage, intraabdominal abscesses, fistulas or intestinal perforations with or without generalized peritonitis. In the Modified Hinchey Classification uncomplicated acute diverticulitis, would belong to stages 0 and Ia.

PHYSIOPATHOLOGY

Colonic diverticula appear more often in the descending and sigmoid colon. They are actually pseudo-diverticula (out-pouching) of the mucosa from the lumen of the colon through the muscularis and adventitia. They usually occur at those points where blood vessels enter the wall of the colon from the mesocolon. Diverticula in the right colon are true diverticular as they include all of the layers of the wall and are usually solitary. On the other hand, in the left colon they are usually multiple and are composed of only mucosa and submucosa.

It has been classically considered that diverticula formed in these weak spots in the colonic wall are due to an increased intraluminal pressure in patients who have a chronic constipation. Histological studies have proven that in patients with diverticular disease, the longitudinal muscle layer of the colonic wall is thicker, and that there is more collagen in both the circular and longitudinal muscle layers. This decreases the elasticity of the wall, making it easier for the mucosa to protrude through it [5].

Table 1. Modified Hinchey Classification

HINCHEY'S CLASSIFICATION	
Stage 0	Clinically mild Diverticulitis
Stage Ia	Pericolic inflammation
Stage Ib	Pericolic or mesocolic ≤4cm abscess
Stage II	Intraabdominal, pelvic, retroperitoneal or abscess distant from primary inflammation
Stage III	Generalized purulent peritonitis
Stage IV	Generalized fecal peritonitis

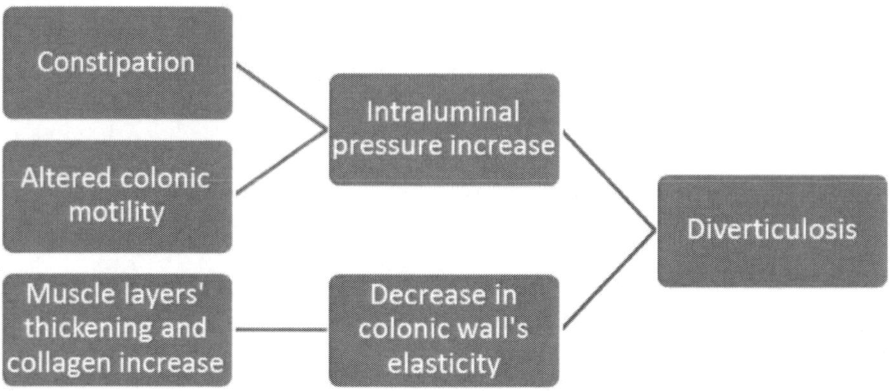

Graph 1. Physiopathology of the diverticular disease.

This structural alteration of the colonic wall allows the formation of small pouches when there is an increase of intraluminal pressure, which is also a consequence of abnormal peristaltic movements. The enteric nervous system is a part of the autonomic nervous system, and the myenteric plexus lies in between the muscle layers of the colonic wall. The signal from the plexus to the myocytes are transmited by the myenteric interstitial cells of cajal. A lower proportion of these types of neurons has been described in patients with diverticular disease.

Based on the theory proposed in 1971 by Painter and Burkitt that a low fiber diet was the cause of the increased intraluminal pressure in the colon and consequently the cause for the development of diverticula, it has been speculated and accepted for decades that these pouches were occupied by feces or food, such as seeds or nuts. This would create an environment for local bacterial overgrowth and later micro-perforation, justifying the need of broad spectrum antibiotics when treating acute diverticulitis [6]. There are other physiopathological theories being currently studied to explain the origin of this inflammation, even in those cases in which there are recurrences in spite of long treatments with bro z ad spectrum antibiotics.

There are several studies that identify environmental factors and certain behaviors as precipitant factors to develop complications of a diverticular disease. These include;

- The absence of fiber in a diet has proven to be a cause of an altered intestinal habit and the development of diverticula and pseudodiverticula. It is also usually associated with a diet high in red meat. A fiber-rich diet that also includes seeds (such as the long time forbidden walnuts or corn) is considered a protective factor for the development of acute diverticulitis [7].
- Low levels of vitamin D, associated to low level of exposure to sunlight, have also been studied as risk factor for the development of complicated acute diverticulitis [8].
- Sedentary lifestyle, along with a high body mass index, has been associated with a higher incidence of this disease [9].
- Multiple studies associate smoking with complicated acute diverticulitis and diverticular hemorrhage [10].
- Chronic administration of certain drugs, such as NSAIDs or corticoids, has an influence in both the incidence and severity of acute diverticulitis [11].

Studies performed on twins have proven a higher relative risk when one of the siblings has been previously affected [12]. A certain hereditary predisposition as part of the origin of the disease can be deduced.

Certain local immunological alterations have been described in these patients, such as an increased number of activated macrophages in the colonic wall and a high genetic expression of pro-inflammatory cytokines (TNF-α, IL-6 and adipokines) [13]. A colonoscopy showing signs compatible with persistent inflammation indicate a higher risk for recurrences.

Currently, the role of the intestinal flora in the development of symptoms of a diverticular disease is doubtful, in spite of the published literature defending this factor as an important one to be taken into consideration. When analyzing the fecal matter of patients with acute diverticulitis (AD), higher proportions of the group Proteobacteria [14], as well as several different kinds of yeasts, were found. A lower proportion of the colonic microbiota with an anti-inflammatory potential, such as Clostridium, Fusobacterium and Lactobacillaceae, have also been described [15]. This imbalance in the bacterial flora of the colon could cause a certain degree of chronic inflammation that could affect and alter the local neuronal cells. This would affect the colonic motility, causing bowel distension and the associated symptoms [16].

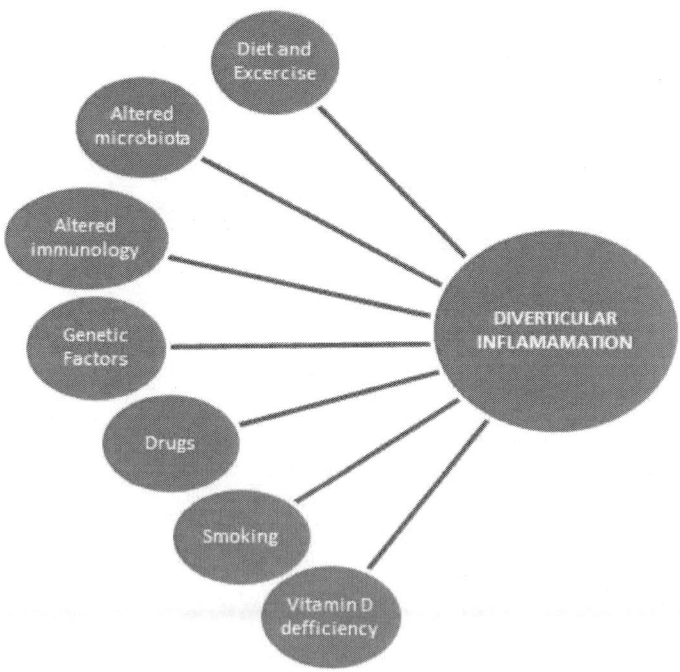
Diet and Excercise
Altered microbiota
Altered immunology
Genetic Factors
Drugs
Smoking
Vitamin D defficiency
DIVERTICULAR INFLAMAMATION

Graph 2. Risk factors for developing complications of diverticular disease.

TREATMENT

Acute diverticulitis includes a range of clinical situations that require a choice between a surgical or a non-surgical conservative management. This choice is made in the acute manifestation and during the follow up [17]. Experts are not able to reach to a consensus; most studies conclude that more trials are needed, whose results might allow creating a series of recommendations based on high-level evidence.

Classical treatment for acute diverticulitis includes the use of broad spectrum antibiotics, either intravenous or oral, analgesia and rest to the digestive tract with a soft or low-residue diet. Multiple trials have proven that this management is not free of persistent and recurrent disease. This fact has been proven in both the milder forms of the disease and in those with more severe situations, in which the management also includes percutaneous drainage of intraabdominal abscesses or even intestinal resections in the most severe cases [18].

During the past decade, conservative management has proven to be safe, without showing a worse evolution of the disease in these patients. Therefore, nowadays in most of the Centers an outpatient management of the non-complicated forms of the disease (stages 0 and Ia of the Modified Hinchey Classification) is being commonly followed [19]. Laparoscopic lavage is also an accepted therapeutical option performed by colorectal surgeons [20]. Primary anastomosis after colonic resection is an another surgical option, where the individual situation of the patient and the risk factors for the anastomotic leak have to been taken into account [21].

Guidelines for management of acute diverticulitis are different in the different western countries [22], making it difficult to establish clear general guidelines for such a prevalent disease. The latest guidelines of The Association of Coloproctology of Great Britain and Ireland recommend routine use of antibiotics for at least a week; however, current guidelines by Dutch, Italian and Danish coloproctological societies' do not recommend this management for uncomplicated cases of acute diverticulitis [23-26]. They have suggested these recommendations independently from one another.

Regarding the non-complicated forms of the disease, the different Societies only agree in the recommendations given for the outpatient management in those patients with no comorbidities. The general use of antibiotics, dietary recommendations and fiber supplements (or, at least, a high-fiber diet) are controversial and each guide gives different indications on the matter [22].

Several studies and revisions have been conducted examining the use of fiber, Rifaximin, Mesalazine and probiotics in primary and secondary prevention, as well as in treatment, in uncomplicated acute diverticulitis. Following is the role played by all these elements in the management of acute diverticulitis.

- Fiber: It is vegetable component consisting of polysaccharides and lignin. It is highly resistant to the hydrolysis of human digestive enzymes. It can be classified into soluble (it slows the intestinal transit) and insoluble (it stimulates the intestinal transit) fiber. It has an important role in maintaining the gut microbiota. It gives consistency to fecal matter and favors intestinal transit. It also reduces intestinal absorption of cholesterol, glucose and biliary acids.
- Rifaximin: It is a byproduct of Rifamycin. This broad spectrum antibiotic is active against gram-positive, gram-negative and anaerobic bacteria. Its intestinal absorption rate is very low, less than 1%, which allows a high concentration in the colonic lumen without the presence of drug in the blood stream. This allows avoiding drug resistances in non-enteric pathogens. Its mechanism of action is by inhibiting the bacterial RNA synthesis by binding to the RNA-polymerase dependent of DNA. On an intestinal level, it prevents bacterial overgrowth, reduces the activity rate of the intestinal flora by acting on species such as Lactobacillus species and Bifidobacterium species. It increases the fecal bolus and has an anti-inflammatory effect as well [27].
- Mesalazine (5-aminisalicylic acid or 5-ASA): It is a local anti-inflammatory drug. Its active metabolite, the N-acetyl-5-ASA, is

responsible for its intestinal effect. Its mechanism of action is not yet well known, but does have an anti-inflammatory effect by inhibiting the synthesis of leukotrienes (specially the leukotriene B4 or LTB4), prostaglandins and cytokines (IL-1). It also has an antioxidant effect by capturing oxygen free-radicals and thus modifies the intraluminal pH and selectively modulates bacterial growth [28]. It has a very low absorption rate of around 25% after oral administration and about 15% after rectal administration. Its half-life varies between 0.5 and 1.5 hours, and the absorbed proportion is excreted by kidneys.

- Probiotics: They are certain kinds of food or supplements containing living microorganisms that can maintain or even improve the intestine's normal microbiota. This microbiota can be altered in patients with diverticular disease due to colonic stasis. A balanced microbiota has an anti-inflammatory effect by inhibiting the secretion of pro-inflammatory cytokines, and improves the intestinal defenses by increasing local IgA secretion [29]. They also prevent bacterial overgrowth, and have influence on the metabolism of different pathogens by interfering their development as these "good" bacteria compete with them for nutrition.

Multiple studies have been performed till date comparing the classical management using broad spectrum antibiotics with a more conservative treatment based on use of analgesics and a relative digestive rest, with a liquid diet first and a soft diet afterwards. The first randomized study was the AVOD (Antibiotika Vid Okomplicerad Divertikulit) study published in 2012 [30], showing promising initial conclusions. This multicenter study, with over 600 patients, randomized the patients into two groups. One group was put on a classical treatment using antibiotics, the other with only digestive rest and analgesia. On comparing both the complication rate (perforation and abscess formation) and the recurrence rate, no statistically significant difference was found between the two groups. This study concludes that the use of antibiotics in mild cases of diverticular disease does not accelerate the recovery, nor it reduces the risk for complications and recurrences. Therefore, it suggests that antibiotics should be reserved only for the more severe cases of the disease.

In the past years, different papers have been published regarding studies performed in this particular field. These studies showed great variability, ranging from series of cases to new randomized clinical trials. Recently at least four meta-analyses have been published comparing these trials, three of which are pending publication when this chapter was edited [31-34]. All of them prove that treating uncomplicated acute diverticulitis as outpatients and not including broad spectrum antibiotics does not have worse results than the classical management. These results come from comparing complication rates (abscess formation and perforation), disease persistence (defined by a new admittance or consultation in the first 30 days after diagnosis), recurrence rate (new episode within the first month after diagnosis), need for surgical treatment and mortality.

A multicenter controlled randomized trial is currently taking place in Europe whose objective is to gather the largest series of patients studied to this day, comparing both lines of treatment [35].

Regarding the drugs aforementioned, varied results can be found. With the information at hand, no formal recommendations have been made in any of the recently published guidelines.

- Fiber and diet: Although results vary between different randomized controlled studies, a high fiber intake is still routinely recommended. This fiber can be obtained from diet and from soluble fiber supplements [36]. These recommendations are based on low level evidence.
- Rifaximin: Several studies have been conducted comparing placebo versus a combination of Rifaximin and fiber supplements. Two recent reviews prove that this combination is an effective treatment in the milder cases of the disease and also in preventing recurrences of acute cases in those patients who have previously had episodes of uncomplicated acute diverticulitis [37]. This treatment is more common in European countries such as Denmark and Italy, where the use of Rifaximin with fiber is recommended. In other countries,

such as Germany and United States, its systemic use is not recommended. The recommended dose of Rifaximin is 400mg/24h for one week per month associated with high amounts of fiber.

- Mesalazine: This anti-inflammatory drug has proven to be effective when treating uncomplicated acute diverticulitis. It reduces the severity of the symptoms and is also useful in secondary prevention of the disease. In some clinical trials, it has even proven to be more effective than Rifaximin and probiotics. However, the combination of Mesalazine and probiotics has obtained better results in preventing fresh episodes of acute diverticulitis rather than combining Mesalazine with placebo [38]. It seems that a continuous treatment is better than a cyclical one. Dose of Mesalazine varies between 1.6 and 3 gm per day. Its recommendation in different international guidelines varies widely. New clinical trials are needed to increase the statistical power to prove its effectiveness.
- Probiotics: The registered clinical trials that have studied this treatment group have not clarified much about its usefulness when treating the disease, mainly because of its low statistical power and, in many cases, its low theoretical quality. However, the combination of Lactobacillus casei with Mesalazine has obtained the best results when used for secondary prevention of the disease [38].

Therapeutical Strategies: Current Indications

Although colonic diverticulosis is very common, especially among older patients, clinical manifestation of diverticular disease is less prevalent than what former data has suggested. Today, it is considered that in patients with colonic diverticulitis, symptoms develop in approximately 5% cases. In spite of what is commonly believed in the scientific community, it has not been possible to clearly establish the association between a low fiber diet or chronic constipation and the development of symptoms. Therefore, the common practice of recommending a high fiber diet as primary prevention can be considered, at least, questionable [36].

Several studies have gathered information about how diverticular disease affects the quality of life of patients. These studies include patients with an active disease and patients with previous episodes of acute diverticulitis, and have shown a wide variety of physical, psychological and social problems among patients.

When treating diverticular disease, the goals are to control the patient's symptoms and also to prevent further recurrent episodes and complications. Amongst the mildest forms of diverticular disease, three different scenarios can be described and the management of each of these situations is described below.

Asymptomatic Diverticular Disease

These are the patients who are diagnosed of having colonic diverticula after a diagnostic procedure has been done for some other reason, but never had any kind of related complication such as inflammation or hemorrhage. They are usually diagnosed after a colonoscopy (where the most common finding is colonic diverticulosis), a CT scan or a sonography performed for some other reasons. This diagnosis is an incidental finding in these diagnostic procedures. Although there is little evidence to support it, different Western guidelines, including the guidelines recommended by American Gastroenterological Association Institute on the Management of Acute Diverticulitis from 2015, recommend a series of healthy habits. These habits include a high fiber diet with low amounts of red meat, avoid smoking, and avoid using NSAIDs, regular physical exercise, maintaining high levels of vitamin D and a proper glycemic control in diabetic patients. Other classical recommendations such as avoid eating nuts or corn have no data to support them and should not be currently suggested.

SYMPTOMATIC UNCOMPLICATED DIVERTICULAR DISEASE (SUDD)

Patients with this condition are those with abdominal pain secondary to the colonic diverticula, but with no inflammation associated to it. This pain usually ceases after a bowel movement or after passing gas. It can also be associated with an altered intestinal transit, including either constipation or diarrhea. No alterations are found on a blood test, and the main differential diagnosis should be made with irritable bowel syndrome, since both share several clinical characteristics. Perhaps, the localization of the pain could help in this differential diagnosis, since patients with irritable bowel syndrome usually have a generalized abdominal pain and patients with Symptomatic uncomplicated diverticular disease typically locate the pain in the left iliac fossa.

Given this situation, several guidelines recommend a high fiber diet and Rifaximin at 400mg/12h one week per month to prevent recurrent symptoms and the development of a diverticular inflammation. This treatment has proven to be more effective than simple observation or treatment with placebo. It also seems that treatment with Mesalazine reduces the clinical manifestations of Symptomatic uncomplicated diverticular disease and reduces the incidence of a first episode of acute diverticulitis; nevertheless, it has not proven to be better than the combination of fiber and Rifaximin. Current studies about the role of probiotic agents do not have enough statistical power to be able to recommend its standard use.

Uncomplicated Acute Diverticulitis (UAD)

85% of cases of acute diverticulitis are uncomplicated acute diverticulitis (UAD) and in the Modified Hinchey Classification uncomplicated acute diverticulitis, would belong to stages 0 and Ia. However, no consensus has been reached regarding its treatment in this group of patients. As we have mentioned before, the classical treatment for

UAD included using broad spectrum antibiotics and relative intestinal rest. This management was based on the physiopathological theory that the inflammation was associated with a micro-perforation, and its goal was to avoid the subsequent bacterial translocation that could cause septicemia. The patient could be treated with hospital admission and intravenous antibiotics, or as an outpatient case with oral antibiotics. Antibiotics of choice had to be active against gram positive, gram negative and anaerobic bacteria; thus, the most commonly used antibiotics were a combination of Ciprofloxacin and Metronidazole or Penicillin by-products, such as Amoxicillin/Clavulanic Acid, Piperacillin/Tazobactam or Carbapenems. The duration of these treatments has changed over time, going from 7 to 14 days on the latest guidelines. However outpatient treatment can be considered only in cases with no signs of severe sepsis, with proper oral intake and with an adequate social and family support

Based on current physiopathological theories, routine use of broad spectrum antibiotics in uncomplicated cases of acute diverticulitis does not seem to add any individual benefit to the patient. Moreover, from a collective point of view, it can cause an increase in drug resistances to different classes of antibiotics and the subsequent problems that these resistances imply. This is already happening in different Western countries. Individual complications include unwanted effects such as diarrhea, opportunistic fungal infections (oral and/or vaginal candidiasis), allergic reactions or pseudomembranous colitis (caused by the bacteria Clostridium difficile). Consequently, the latest guidelines for treatment of acute diverticulitis do not recommend standard use of antibiotics in uncomplicated cases and low risk patients (immunocompetent patients without any co-morbidities) [23-26]. Treatment in these cases should be based on analgesic drugs and a soft low-residue diet. Analgesics include NSAIDs, since it has not been proven that they cause a bad evolution during the acute stage of the disease. This treatment can also be carried out as an outpatient treatment with periodical visits to the medical office. Depending on the studies published by different authors, the visits can be carried out every 5 to 30 days.

Recurrences have been described in up to 30% of patients; therefore, treatment of acute diverticulitis must include control over the symptoms in the acute stage and also prevention of recurrences and complications. The latest revisions and meta-analysis describe a higher recurrence rate, but without statistical significance in treatment failure, complications, recurrences, readmission rate, need for surgical treatment or mortality [31].

The main arguments against this management option comes from the selection bias that the studies analyzed in these meta-analysis have. All of these studies include patients with no associated risk factors (immunodepression or associated co-morbidities) and have the mildest forms of the disease (Modified Hinchey Classification 0 and Ia). Although, we must not forget that the current guidelines that recommend this management, only do it in these selected groups of patients. This type of management in more severe stages of disease (Hinchey Ib) requires further studies. There seems to be no physiopathological basis to support avoiding the use of antibiotics in those cases which are associated with sepsis, as happens in all patients with purulent or fecal peritonitis (stages Hinchey III and IV), and in most patients with associated abscesses (Hinchey II).

Table 2. Diverticular Disease's Management

Presentation	Treatment
Divertículos	No treatment needed
Symptomatic uncomplicated diverticular disease (SUDD)	Fiber (diet or supplements) + Rifaximin 400mg/12h, 7 days per month
Uncomplicated Acute Diverticulitis	Liquid diet 24-48 hours followed by soft diet Symptomatic treatment (analgesia) Antibiotics in selected patients (immunodeficiency, previous comorbidities)

CONCLUSION

With the latest advances in the study of the diverticular disease and our better understanding of its physiology, we have been able to create new management strategies. These strategies include restricting the use of antibiotics only to the more severe cases or with patients with risk factors for bad evolution. This line of treatment is safe, as proven by different randomized trials and meta-analyses; furthermore, it does not have a higher incidence of complications when compared with the classical treatment, which includes use of systemic antibiotics.

REFERENCES

[1] Everhart, J. E. & Constance E. Ruhl. (2009). "Burden Of Digestive Diseases In The United States Part II: Lower Gastrointestinal Diseases". *Gastroenterology*, *136* (3), 741-754. doi: 10.1053/j.gastro. 2009.01.015.

[2] Broderick-Villa, G. (2005). "Hospitalization For Acute Diverticulitis Does Not Mandate Routine Elective Colectomy". *Archives Of Surgery*, *140*(6), 576. doi: 10.1001/archsurg.140.6.576.

[3] Strate, L., Modi, R., Cohen, E. & Spiegel, B. (2012). "Diverticular Disease as a Chronic Illness: Evolving Epidemiologic and Clinical Insight"s. *The American Journal of Gastroenterology*, *107*(10), 1486-1493. doi: 10.1038/ajg.2012.194.

[4] Tursi, A., Papa, A. & Danese, S. (2015). "Review article: the pathophysiology and medical management of diverticulosis and diverticular disease of the colon". *Alimentary Pharmacology & Therapeutics*, *42*(6), 664-684. doi: 10.1111/apt.13322.

[5] Hobson, Kristina G, & Patricia L Roberts. (2006). "Etiology And Pathophysiology Of Diverticular Disease". *Clinics In Colon And Rectal Surgery*, *17* (3), 147-153. doi: 10.1055/s-2004-832695.

[6] Painter, N. S. & Burkitt, D. P. (1971). Diverticular disease of the colon: a deficiency disease of Western civilization. *British medical journal, 2*(5759), 450-4.

[7] Korzenik, Joshua R. (2006). “Case Closed?”. *Journal Of Clinical Gastroenterology, 40* (Supplement 3): S112-S116. doi: 10.1097/01. mcg.0000225503.59923.6c.

[8] Nguyen, Geoffrey C. (2011). “Epidemiological Trends And Geographic Variation In Hospital Admissions For Diverticulitis In The United States”. *World Journal Of Gastroenterology, 17* (12), 1600. doi: 10.3748/wjg.v17.i12.1600.

[9] Rosemar, Anders, Ulf Angerås, & Annika Rosengren. (2008). “Body Mass Index And Diverticular Disease: A 28-Year Follow-Up Study In Men”. *Diseases Of The Colon & Rectum, 51* (4), 450-455. doi: 10. 1007/s10350-007-9172-5.

[10] Turunen, P., Wikström, H., Carpelan-Holmström, M., Kairaluoma, P., Kruuna, O. & Scheinin, T. (2010). “Smoking Increases The Incidence Of Complicated Diverticular Disease Of The Sigmoid Colon”. *Scandinavian Journal Of Surgery, 99* (1), 14-17. doi: 10.1177/ 145749691009900104.

[11] Kvasnovsky, C. L., S. Papagrigoriadis, and I. Bjarnason. (2014). “Increased Diverticular Complications With Nonsteriodal Anti-Inflammatory Drugs And Other Medications: A Systematic Review And Meta-Analysis”. *Colorectal Disease, 16* (6), O189-O196. doi: 10. 1111/codi.12516.

[12] Strate, Lisa L., Rune Erichsen, John A. Baron, Jakob Mortensen, Jacob Krabbe Pedersen, Anders H. Riis, Kaare Christensen, and Henrik Toft Sørensen. (2013). “Heritability And Familial Aggregation Of Diverticular Disease: A Population-Based Study Of Twins And Siblings”. *Gastroenterology, 144*(4), 736-742. e1. doi: 10.1053/j. gastro.2012.12.030.

[13] Schieffer, Kathleen M., Christine S. Choi, Scott Emrich, Leonard Harris, Sue Deiling, Dipti M. Karamchandani, Anna Salzberg, Yuka I. Kawasawa, Gregory S. Yochum, & Walter A. Koltun. (2017). “RNA-Seq Implicates Deregulation Of The Immune System In The

Pathogenesis Of Diverticulitis". *American Journal Of Physiology-Gastrointestinal And Liver Physiology*, *313* (3), G277-G284. doi: 10. 1152/ajpgi.00136.2017.

[14] Daniels, L., Budding, A. E., de Korte, N., Eck, A., Bogaards, J. A., Stockmann, H. B., Consten, E. C., Savelkoul, P. H. & Boermeester, M. A. (2014). "Fecal Microbiome Analysis As A Diagnostic Test For Diverticulitis". *European Journal Of Clinical Microbiology & Infectious Diseases*, *33* (11), 1927-1936. doi: 10.1007/s10096-014-2162-3.

[15] Barbara, Giovanni, Eleonora Scaioli, Maria Raffaella Barbaro, Elena Biagi, Luca Laghi, Cesare Cremon, & Giovanni Marasco et al. (2016). "Gut Microbiota, Metabolome And Immune Signatures In Patients With Uncomplicated Diverticular Disease". *Gut*, *66* (7), 1252-1261. doi: 10.1136/gutjnl-2016-312377.

[16] Bassotti, G., Battaglia, E., Deroberto, G., Morelli, A., Tonini, M. & Villanacci, V. (2005). "Alterations In Colonic Motility And Relationship To Pain In Colonic Diverticulosis". *Clinical Gastroenterology And Hepatology*, *3* (3), 248-253. doi: 10.1016/ s1542-3565(04)00614-7.

[17] O'Leary, D. Peter, Noel Lynch, Cillian Clancy, Desmond C. Winter, & Eddie Myers. (2015). "International, Expert-Based, Consensus Statement Regarding The Management Of Acute Diverticulitis". *JAMA Surgery*, *150* (9), 899. doi: 10.1001/jamasurg.2015.1675.

[18] Feingold, Daniel, Scott R. Steele, Sang Lee, Andreas Kaiser, Robin Boushey, W. Donald Buie, & Janice Frederick Rafferty. (2014). "Practice Parameters For The Treatment Of Sigmoid Diverticulitis". *Diseases Of The Colon & Rectum*, *57* (3), 284-294. doi: 10.1097/ dcr.0000000000000075.

[19] Biondo, Sebastiano, Thomas Golda, Esther Kreisler, Eloy Espin, Francesc Vallribera, Fabiola Oteiza, Antonio Codina-Cazador, Marcel Pujadas, & Blas Flor. (2014). "Outpatient Versus Hospitalization Management For Uncomplicated Diverticulitis." *Annals of Surgery*, *259*(1), 38-44. doi: 10.1097/SLA.0b013e3182965a11.

[20] Angenete, E., Bock, D., Rosenberg, J. & Haglind, E. (2016). Laparoscopic lavage is superior to colon resection for perforated purulent diverticulitis-a meta-analysis. *International journal of colorectal disease*, *32*(2), 163-169. doi: 10.1007%2Fs00384-016-2636-0

[21] Reyes-Espejel, L., Ruiz-Campos, M., Correa-Rovelo, J. M. & García-Osogobio, S. (2015). "Sigmoidectomy With Primary Anastomosis For Complicated Diverticulitis". *Revista De Gastroenterología De México (English Edition)*, *80* (4), 255-259. doi: 10.1016/j.rgmxen.2015.07.007.

[22] Galetin, T., Galetin, A., Vestweber, K. H. & Rink, A. D. (2018). "Systematic Review And Comparison Of National And International Guidelines On Diverticular Disease". *International Journal Of Colorectal Disease*, *33* (3), 261-272. doi: 10.1007/s00384-017-2960-z.

[23] Association of Coloproctology of Great Britain and Ireland. Commissioning guide: colonic diverticular disease. https://www.acpgbi.org.uk/content/uploads/2017/02/Commissioning-guide-colonic-diverticular-disease-RCS-2014.pdf.

[24] Andeweg, Caroline S., Irene M. Mulder, Richelle J. F. Felt-Bersma, Annelies Verbon, Gert Jan van der Wilt, Harry van Goor, Johan F. Lange, Jaap Stoker, Marja A. Boermeester, & Robert P. Bleichrodt. (2013). "Guidelines Of Diagnostics And Treatment Of Acute Left-Sided Colonic Diverticulitis". *Digestive Surgery*, *30* (4-6), 278-292. doi: 10.1159/000354035.

[25] Binda, G. A., Cuomo, R., Laghi, A., Nascimbeni, R., Serventi, A., Bellini, D., Gervaz, P. & Annibale, B. (2015). "Practice Parameters For The Treatment Of Colonic Diverticular Disease: Italian Society Of Colon And Rectal Surgery (SICCR) Guidelines". *Techniques In Coloproctology*, *19* (10), 615-626. doi: 10.1007/s10151-015-1370-x.

[26] Andersen, J. C., Bundgaard, L., Elbrønd, H., Laurberg, S., Walker, L. R. & Støvring, J. (2012). Danish Surgical Society. Danish national guidelines for treatment of diverticular disease. *Danish Medical Journal*, *59*, C4453.

[27] Scarpignato, Carmelo, & Iva Pelosini. (2005). "Rifaximin, A Poorly Absorbed Antibiotic: Pharmacology And Clinical Potential". *Chemotherapy*, *51* (1), 36-66. doi: 10.1159/000081990.

[28] Gatta, Luigi, Nimish Vakil, Dino Vaira, Alberto Pilotto, Margherita Curlo, Giuseppe Comparato, & Gioacchino Leandro et al. (2010). "Efficacy Of 5-ASA In The Treatment Of Colonic Diverticular Disease". *Journal Of Clinical Gastroenterology*, *44* (2), 113-119. doi: 10.1097/mcg.0b013e3181a15864.

[29] Narula, Neeraj, & John K Marshall. (2010). "Role Of Probiotics In Management Of Diverticular Disease". *Journal Of Gastroenterology And Hepatology*, *25* (12), 1827-1830. doi: 10.1111/j.1440-1746.2010. 06444.x.

[30] Chabok, A., Påhlman, L., Hjern, F., Haapaniemi, S. & Smedh, K. (2012). "Randomized Clinical Trial Of Antibiotics In Acute Uncomplicated Diverticulitis". *British Journal Of Surgery*, *99* (4), 532-539. doi: 10.1002/bjs.8688.

[31] Emile, S. H., Elfeki, H., Sakr, A. & Shalaby, M. (2018). "Management Of Acute Uncomplicated Diverticulitis Without Antibiotics: A Systematic Review, Meta-Analysis, And Meta-Regression Of Predictors Of Treatment Failure". *Techniques In Coloproctology*, *22* (7), 499-509. doi: 10.1007/s10151-018-1817-y.

[32] Mege, Diane, & Heather Yeo. (2019). "Meta-Analyses Of Current Strategies To Treat Uncomplicated Diverticulitis". *Diseases Of The Colon & Rectum*, *62* (3), 371-378. doi: 10.1097/dcr. 0000000000001295.

[33] Desai, M., Fathallah, J., Nutalapati, V. & Saligram, S. (2019). Antibiotics Versus No Antibiotics for Acute Uncomplicated Diverticulitis. *Diseases of the Colon & Rectum*, *62*, 00–00 (Epub ahead of print). doi: 10.7759%2Fcureus.1250.

[34] Au, Stephanie, & Emad H. Aly. (2019)."Treatment Of Uncomplicated Acute Diverticulitis Without Antibiotics". *Diseases Of The Colon & Rectum*, *1*. doi: 10.1097/dcr.0000000000001330. (Epub ahead of print).

[35] Mora Lopez, Laura, Neus Ruiz-Edo, Sheila Serra Pla, Anna Pallisera Llovera, Salvador Navarro Soto, & Xavier Serra-Aracil. (2017). "Multicentre, Controlled, Randomized Clinical Trial To Compare The Efficacy And Safety Of Ambulatory Treatment Of Mild Acute Diverticulitis Without Antibiotics With The Standard Treatment With Antibiotics". *International Journal Of Colorectal Disease*, *32* (10): 1509-1516. doi: 10.1007/s00384-017-2879-4.

[36] Peery, Anne F., Patrick R. Barrett, Doyun Park, Albert J. Rogers, Joseph A. Galanko, Christopher F. Martin, & Robert S. Sandler. (2012). "A High-Fiber Diet Does Not Protect Against Asymptomatic Diverticulosis". *Gastroenterology*, *142* (2), 266-272. e1. doi: 10.1053/ j.gastro.2011.10.035.

[37] Bianchi, M., Festa, V., Moretti, A., Ciaco, A., Mangone, M., Tornatore, V. & Dezi, A., et al. (2011). "Meta-Analysis: Long-Term Therapy With Rifaximin In The Management Of Uncomplicated Diverticular Disease". *Alimentary Pharmacology & Therapeutics*, *33* (8), 902-910. doi: 10.1111/j.1365-2036.2011.04606.x.

[38] Tursi, A., Brandimarte, G., Elisei, W., Picchio, M., Forti, G., Pianese, G. & Rodino, S., et al. (2013). "Randomised Clinical Trial: Mesalazine And/Or Probiotics In Maintaining Remission Of Symptomatic Uncomplicated Diverticular Disease - A Double-Blind, Randomised, Placebo-Controlled Study". *Alimentary Pharmacology & Therapeutics*, *38* (7), 741-751. doi: 10.1111/apt.12463.

In: Diverticulitis: Diagnosis and Treatment ISBN: 978-1-53618-081-7
Editors: Shams-ul-Bari et al.

Chapter 4

SURGICAL TREATMENT OF DIVERTICULITIS

Abdelghaffar Salous[1], MD, PhD, JoAnn Coleman[1], DNP and Vanita Ahuja[2,*], MD, MPH, MBA

[1]Department of General Surgery,
Sinai Hospital of Baltimore, Baltimore, MD, USA
[2]Department of Surgery, Yale School of Medicine, New Haven, CT, USA

ABSTRACT

Acute diverticulitis is a common disease in the western world [1]. A recent epidemiological analysis by our group showed a rise both in the incidence and hospitalization for acute diverticulitis, independent of race [2]. Symptomatic diverticulitis represents a fraction of diverticular disease. Hinchey I and II acute diverticulitis are treated with bowel rest, antibiotics, and percutaneous drainage (if indicated) [3], while acute surgical intervention is reserved for Hinchey class III and class IV diverticulitis that present with perforation, peritonitis, sepsis, and failure of non-operative treatment [4]. Traditionally, Hinchey class III and IV diverticulitis has been a clear indication for acute surgical intervention [4, 5]. The significant morbidity associated with urgent colectomy has led to a shift to non-

* Corresponding Author's Email: Vanita.ahuja@yale.edu.

operative management in non-toxic appearing patients [5]. However, approximately 1 in 5 patients are hospitalized with recurrent acute diverticulitis and eventually undergo surgical intervention [6]. Although percutaneous drainage for Hinchey class I and II diverticulitis is well accepted, the rate of recurrence in this subset of patients in some studies is three folds higher than patients who underwent elective resection [7]. Grading systems (mainly based on CT imaging findings) have been used to quantify such risk and guide decision-making. Interestingly, the severity of the episode, rather than age, was a better determinant of recurrence that ranged between 10%-35% [7]. The contribution of patient-specific risk factors to recurrence/severity of disease has not been elucidated, but the presence of comorbidities renders surgical decision making more difficult as those sicker patients are susceptible to both the complications of the disease (severity, perforation) and the complications of the treatment (colectomy) [8]. Our group developed and validated a scoring system to quantify the risk of Hartmann's reversal [9]. Overall, the bulk of evidence from recent studies weighs in favor of an individualized approach for patients considering elective colectomy. From a technical approach, laparoscopic colectomy has not been inferior to open resection with respect to complications and, in fact, the laparoscopic approach resulted in better short-term outcomes in several studies [10]. The high morbidity associated with Hartmann's procedure increased interest in maintaining intestinal continuity and gave rise to performing partial colectomy with primary anastomosis and proximal diversion or consideration of peritoneal lavage as a damage control operation [11, 12]. Data on peritoneal lavage is fairly limited and subject to significant selection bias [13]. Surgical intervention continues to be an important modality in the treatment of acute diverticulitis, with a steady transition toward less invasive interventions and optimization of medical therapy [14]. Ongoing assessment of the long-term effects of the surgical modalities is still needed to refine surgical management of this disease.

Keywords: diverticulitis, Hinchey classification, Hartmann's procedure, fast track recovery, surgery

INTRODUCTION

Colonic diverticular disease is a term that encompasses several manifestations involving colonic diverticula-a pouch-like protrusion in which the mucosal and submucosal layers herniate through the muscular layer of the colonic wall. The prevalence of diverticular disease increases with age and approximately 60% of Americans develop diverticula by age 60 [15]. While the majority (70-80%) of patients remain asymptomatic, approximately 5-15% of patients with diverticular disease experience diverticular bleeding [16, 17] and 4-5% experience diverticulitis [18-20]. Of those patients with diverticulitis, 80% have an uncomplicated form of the disease and 15-20% proceed to have complicated manifestations, namely abscess, perforation, fistula, obstruction, or recurrence [21].

This chapter reviews the pathophysiology, epidemiology, diagnosis, and classification systems of complicated diverticulitis in relation to surgical management. A review of surgical approaches, timing of surgery, outcomes, follow-up, and development of a personalized surgical approach to each patient is presented in light of the updated guidelines of the American Society of Colorectal Surgery (ASCRS) published in 2014, and the American Gastroenterological Association (AGA) published in 2015.

PATHOPHYSIOLOGY

The pathophysiology of diverticulitis is not completely understood. Long standing, unproven theories suggested diverticulitis resulted from an inflammatory process characterized by the sequence of diverticular obstruction, increased intraluminal pressure, ischemia, necrosis, and perforation [22]. This theory explains the traditional widespread belief that patients should avoid nuts and seeds, which was later debunked by multiple studies that showed consumption of these does not increase the risk of diverticulitis [23]. Additionally, the theory of acute inflammation has been questioned, as the use of antibiotics in uncomplicated acute diverticulitis was not shown to accelerate recovery or prevent recurrence or complications [24, 25]. Growing evidence suggests a complex chronic inflammation process with multiple interplay including risk factors [26]. Several studies documented increased risk of diverticulitis with western diet [27], obesity [28], use of NSAIDs [29], and smoking [30-32]. Conversely, dietary fiber intake [32] and adherence to a healthy lifestyle decreased this risk [33].

Modifying these factors in the acute setting is not pragmatic, especially with respect to patients requiring surgical intervention. Educating patients on these factors is important to reduce the long-term burden of disease and the potential need for future surgical intervention.

EPIDEMIOLOGY

Colonic diverticulitis is associated with a heavy economic burden reflected by the increase in admissions and operations, especially for younger patients [1]. In 2009, diverticulitis ranked third among gastrointestinal diagnoses, accounted for 200,000 discharges, and exceeded $2 billion dollars. Recent analysis of data from the National Inpatient Sample (NIS) from 2002 to 2007 revealed an increased incidence of diverticulitis, hospital admission rate, and proportion of younger patients aged 18-49 affected by diverticulitis [21].

Several risk factors and comorbidities are noteworthy when evaluating patients. Diverticulitis is more common in men than women until the fifth decade when it becomes equal [21]. Hospitalization has been steadily increasing over time across all races but is greatest in whites (Caucasians) (62/100,000), followed by Native Americans (50/100,000), African Americans and Hispanics (30/100,000), and lowest in Asians (10/100,00) [34]. Asian patients have a higher incidence of cecal/right colonic diverticulitis [35]. Living in urban areas [36] and a lower socioeconomic status [37] were associated with higher likelihood for hospitalization. Although diverticulitis is more common in industrialized nations, the possibility of hospitalization for immigrants suffering from diverticulitis increases over time, reflecting the risk conferred by the Western lifestyle [38]. When obtaining a patient's medical history, it is important to inquire about immunosuppression. Theoretically, impaired healing may contribute to perforation and/or mask the signs and symptoms of the inflammatory response. This may account for increased disease severity, likelihood for surgical intervention, and poorer outcomes [38]. In recognition of these epidemiologic trends, various clinical presentations of diverticulitis, as discussed above, and increasing comorbidities in the patient population, make surgical intervention not only warranted but also challenging.

DIAGNOSIS

The triad of left lower quadrant abdominal pain, fever, and leukocytosis is the most common clinical presentation of acute diverticulitis [39]. Abdominal pain is the most common complaint followed by nausea, vomiting, fevers, and alteration in bowel habits [26]. Pain may be suprapubic in a redundant sigmoid colon and predominantly right-sided in Asian patients [40]. A focused history and physical examination should specifically inquire about fecaluria and pneumaturia, which may be present with a colovesical fistula. Diagnostic evaluation should include a digital rectal exam to check for palpable masses and bleeding.

The differential diagnosis of acute diverticulitis includes urinary tract infections, symptomatic nephrolithiasis, bowel obstruction, inflammatory bowel disease (IBD), ischemic bowel, neoplastic disease, and gynecologic disorders. Initial diagnostic workup should also include a complete blood count, urinalysis, and an abdominal radiograph [41].

The diagnostic accuracy of diverticulitis based on clinical assessment alone has been reported as low, with sensitivity of 64%-68%. Computed tomography (CT) imaging with intravenous (IV) and luminal contrast had the highest sensitivity of 95% and specificity of 96%. Ultrasound (US) sensitivity and specificity were 90%. Magnetic resonance imaging had the highest sensitivity of 98% but a low specificity range of 70-78%. Contrast enemas had the lowest sensitivity of 80% [41]. Beyond its diagnostic accuracy, CT imaging has the added benefit of grading the severity of disease which correlated with both short and long term complications [42]. Ultrasound is more widely used in Europe. Additional limitations to using US imaging are operator dependence, patient tenderness and obesity [43]. Abdominal radiographs have the least utility as they show nonspecific findings in up to half the patients with diverticulitis. However, an erect radiograph may show pneumoperitoneum [44]. CT imaging is the gold standard for evaluation of diverticulitis and most informative for guiding operative vs non-operative management of patients afflicted with this disease.

Hinchey Classification

Dr. E. John Hinchey first described complicated diverticulitis in 1978 to assess the degree of peritoneal contamination from perforation, as listed below [45]. Several (6-7) additional modified classifications [46] ensued but the original Hinchey classification (described below) remains widely used today. Hinchey classification is useful to physicians, especially surgeons, to triage patients to the proper therapy: medical management with antibiotics, percutaneous drainage, or urgent laparotomy. Currently, the classification is based on CT imaging results.

Stage I – Peri-colic or mesenteric abscess
Stage II – Walled-off pelvic abscess
Stage III – Generalized purulent peritonitis
Stage IV – Generalized fecal peritonitis

All patients benefit from medical management (bowel rest, intravenous resuscitation, and antibiotics). One of the limitations of this classification is differentiating between stage III and stage IV on CT imaging. However, the recommended management remains the same for both classes, namely emergent laparotomy [7].

TREATMENT

A systematic approach to evaluating and treating patients with diverticulitis relies on performing a thorough history and physical examination, review of laboratory values, and careful interpretation of imaging findings by the operating surgeon. The approach to this process relies on evaluating the need for hospitalization, weighing operative and non-operative management measures, and the proper timing of operative intervention (emergent vs urgent vs elective). Medical management should be used whenever possible with the aim of converting an emergent/urgent operation to an elective operation.

A simplified approach is illustrated in Figure 1 with a detailed discussion to follow. After confirming the diagnosis of acute diverticulitis, the need for hospitalization is assessed. Patients with uncomplicated diverticulitis (Hinchey class 0) who tolerate oral intake, whose pain is controlled, and otherwise have met no indication for hospitalization, can be discharged and followed as an outpatient for medical management and elective surgical evaluation (if needed).

- Patients that meet criteria for hospitalization, including those who failed outpatient treatment, should be admitted and given a trial of non-operative management (bowel rest, intravenous (IV) antibiotics, pain control, and IV fluids). After repeat evaluation and depending on their progression, these patients are triaged to either urgent or elective surgical intervention. An exception to this rule is high-risk (immunocompromised) patients with uncomplicated disease who should proceed to urgent surgical intervention.
- Patients with contained perforation (Hinchey class I, II) should be offered medical treatment (bowel rest, IV pain control, IV antibiotics) and undergo percutaneous drainage. Their response to this combination then dictates urgent vs elective intervention. This group also includes the subset of patients who simultaneously fail treatment with antibiotics and are not amenable to percutaneous drainage, thereby necessitating urgent surgical intervention.
- Patients with frank perforation (Hinchey class III, IV) must undergo emergent surgery.
- Patients with the long-term sequalae of disease (fistula, stricture) are referred for elective surgery.

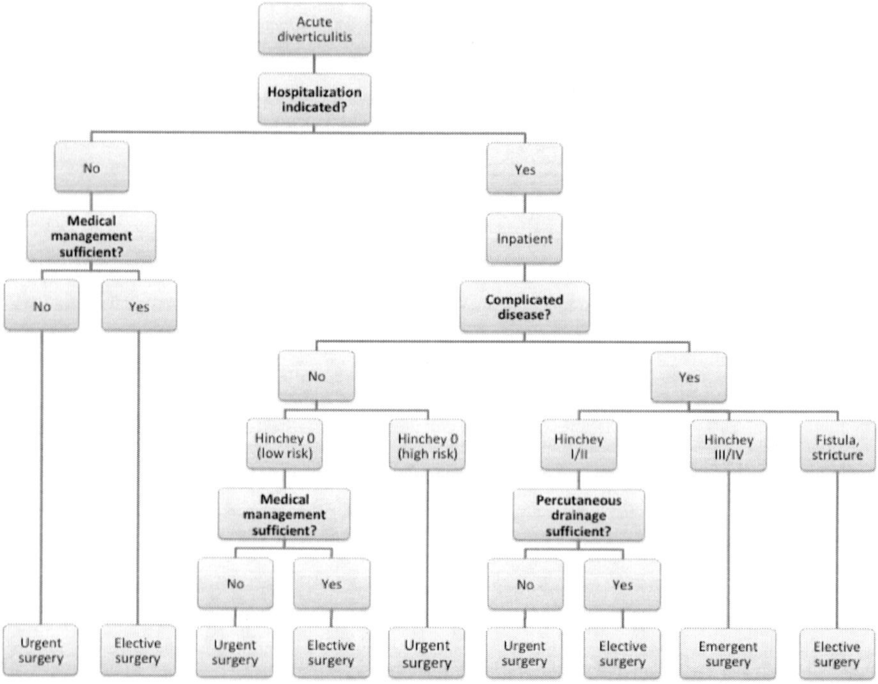

Figure 1. Algorithm for surgical management of acute diverticulitis.

Uncomplicated Diverticulitis (Hinchey Class 0)

Patient selection for surgical intervention is perhaps the most challenging decision for the operating surgeon. First, treatment for patients in this class has been shifting from inpatient to outpatient settings; the DIVER trial showed outpatient and inpatient treatment resulted in similar failure rates and quality of life [47]. Two European randomized clinical trials, Antibiotika Vid Okomplicerad Divertikulit (AVOD) [25] and DIABOLO [24], demonstrated evidence supporting less need for antibiotics and concluded no difference in time to recovery, complications, or recurrence. However, in the latter group, longer follow-up revealed a higher proportion of patients in the placebo group underwent elective surgery secondary to obstruction and recurrence of diverticulitis. Current practice guidelines in the United States continue to recommend antibiotics for this group of patients, citing the lack of long-term data [48]. The adoption of this measure, however, should heighten the operating surgeon's suspicion for the possible need for surgical intervention in these patients.

Hospital admission is indicated for uncomplicated diverticulitis patients with high risk factors including advanced age, intolerance of oral intake, immunosuppression, significant comorbidities, failed outpatient treatment, high fevers (>102.5°F/39°C), severe abdominal pain, diffuse peritonitis, significant leukocytosis, sepsis, and noncompliance/ unreliability [42]. The surgical team should continue to monitor these high-risk patients with uncomplicated diverticulitis until resolution of symptoms, as non-operative treatment failure warrants urgent surgical intervention. Performing serial abdominal examinations, trending markers of infection/inflammation, and repeating imaging studies aid in this assessment. Depending on their progression, these patients may be triaged to inpatient or elective surgical intervention.

Several misconceptions surround the practice of elective sigmoidectomy for patients with uncomplicated diverticulitis. First, the practice of elective colectomy to prevent future recurrences requiring stoma formation is no longer recommended by ASCRS [42]. Previously, the number of recurrences was an indication for surgical intervention, but more recently, research findings demonstrated no increase in morbidity or mortality between patients who have more than two episodes of diverticulitis compared to those with fewer episodes, bolstering the notion that acute diverticulitis is not a progressive disease [49]. Additionally, the decrease in surgical treatment was not associated with an increase in complicated diverticulitis, including perforations [5].

The second common misconception that younger patients suffer worse outcomes of diverticulitis, and consequently need surgical intervention, has been debunked [50]. Studies also showed similar virulence of disease regardless of age, and comparable rates of resection and stoma formation [51]. Contrary to previous reports, the increased morbidity, mortality, and stoma formation is associated with older patients undergoing elective surgical resection for acute diverticulitis [52].

Third, up to 25% of patients reported persistent symptoms, including painful constipation, painful abdominal distension, abdominal cramps, and frequent painful diarrhea following sigmoidectomy for diverticulitis [53, 54]. Moreover, as many as 15% of patients continue to have recurrence after sigmoidectomy [55]. In contrast, the recent multicenter randomized controlled trial showed that elective sigmoidectomy results in a better quality of life than conservative management in patients with diverticulitis [56]. Currently, the preponderance of evidence and recommendations by the ASCRS urge caution with respect to surgical intervention for uncomplicated diverticulitis in otherwise healthy patients.

Conversely, two groups of patient populations with a first attack of uncomplicated diverticulitis demonstrated the surgeon should have a low threshold for elective intervention. The first group is post-hysterectomy patients with acute diverticulitis. This group was found to have an increased rate of pelvic fistula formation following an attack of diverticulitis [57]. The second group encompasses patients on long-term corticosteroids or immunosuppressive medications (transplant recipients), patients with chronic renal failure, and those with collagen vascular disease [58]. The weakened immune response in these patients predisposes them to fail medical management and require emergency surgery [59]. The risks of surgery and failure to alleviate symptoms should also be considered in these patients and balanced with the benefits of surgical treatment.

Complicated Diverticulitis (Hinchey Class I-IV)

Hinchey stages I, II are currently treated with percutaneous drainage or primarily with intravenous antibiotics if the abscess is too small or not amenable to percutaneous drainage [60]. The widespread use of percutaneous drainage allowed the majority of patients to avoid urgent colectomy and undergo an elective one-stage procedure [61], especially since recurrence in this patient population approaches 40% [7]. However, if the hospitalized patient continues to deteriorate or fails to improve with antibiotics and percutaneous drainage, urgent surgical intervention is indicated [3]. This underscores the importance of regular examination of these patients by the surgical team to reassess the need for surgical intervention, even after percutaneous drainage is performed. Hinchey III, IV disease, which consists of frank perforation and generalized peritonitis, is a clear indication for emergent surgical intervention. For these stages, a Hartmann's procedure is performed [42]. Several trials have investigated sigmoidectomy with primary anastomosis protected by a diverting ostomy, challenging the traditional Hartmann's procedure. A multicenter randomized controlled trial of Hinchey III/IV patients showed no difference in morbidity and mortality between the two patient groups, as well as a significantly increased reversal rate in the diverting ileostomy group. A notable decrease in serious complications, operating time, hospital stay, and in-hospital costs was also noted [62]. Another study echoed these findings, showing similar morbidity and mortality profile between the two procedures and a significantly increased stoma closure rate in the protective ileostomy group [63]. However, it is likely that more studies are required before this procedure can be widely recommended for patients with class III/IV Hinchey diverticulitis.

Other Manifestations of Complicated Diverticulitis

Chronic sequalae of diverticulitis include smoldering diverticulitis, fistulas, and strictures. These patients usually have minimal contamination and would benefit from a one-step procedure that involves definitive resection of the diseased segment and primary colorectal anastomosis without a protective ostomy [46, 64].

Operative Techniques

The three main goals of surgical management for diverticulitis are resection of the diseased segment, restoring intestinal continuity, and improving the quality of life (avoidance of ostomy). The reconstruction phase of surgery depends on the degree of contamination and guides whether fecal diversion is performed. The surgical techniques are classified into one-stage, two-stage (resection and diversion, re-establish continuity), three-stage procedures (drainage and diversion, resection, ostomy closure), and laparoscopic lavage [65].

The choice of the appropriate procedure is surgeon and patient dependent, especially with respect to fecal diversion. All factors being equal, the degree of contamination can be used as a rough guide for procedure selection by the operating surgeon.

Elective Surgery (One-Stage Procedure)

In the one-stage operation, sigmoidectomy is performed and followed by primary colorectal anastomosis during the same procedure. The one-stage operation should be used for patients who have minimal contamination, an indication for elective surgery (see Figure 1), and the ability to tolerate a bowel preparation. This procedure is contraindicated for patients with factors that could lead to anastomotic complications. These factors include major medical comorbidities, poor nutritional status, immunosuppression, and immobility. This procedure is also most appropriate for patients with chronic diverticulitis and its sequalae such as strictures and fistulas.

Urgent Surgery (Two-Stage Procedure)

The two-stage procedure has two variants. In one variant, the first stage involves sigmoidectomy with primary colorectal anastomosis and creation of a diverting ileostomy/colostomy; the second stage involves reversing the diverting ostomy. Patients with localized or minimal contamination, those with Hinchey class I/II diverticulitis, should undergo primary anastomosis following resection, with an optional diverting protective loop ileostomy [66].

Emergent Surgery (Two-Stage and Three-Stage Procedures)

The other variant of the two-phase operation, classically known as Hartmann's procedure, involves sigmoidectomy and creation of an end colostomy in the first stage. The second stage of this two-phase operation involves takedown of the end colostomy and re-establishing colorectal continuity [67]. Hartmann's procedure is indicated for patients with diffuse contamination. The rationale for creating the colostomy (as opposed to primary anastomosis) is that infection, inflammation, and shock will compromise healing of a descending colorectal anastomosis [68]. Two European randomized controlled trials on primary anastomosis vs Hartmann's procedure showed post-operative complications, mortality, and stoma-free survival after a Hartmann's procedure which were equivalent or inferior to colectomy with a primary anastomosis with or without a diverting loop ileostomy [24, 62].

The three-stage procedure, described by Mayo, is rarely performed and reserved for patients with severe sepsis. The first stage involves drainage without resection and construction of a proximal diverting ostomy. In the second stage, the diseased segment is resected and a primary anastomosis is performed. In the third stage, the diverting ostomy is closed [65].

Finally, laparoscopic lavage is an alternative approach that represents operative treatment/therapy without resection of the disease focus. Three clinical trials (SCANDIV, LOLA, and DILALA) evaluated this approach and had significant heterogeneity and conflicting results. It is currently considered inappropriate [42].

Preoperative/Perioperative Considerations

Preoperative Colonoscopy

Patients with an attack of acute diverticulitis, with colonic wall thickening on CT should undergo endoscopic evaluation 6-8 weeks after the symptoms completely resolve [42]. The goal is to exclude colonic ischemia, inflammatory bowel disease, and, most importantly, neoplasia [72]. The prevalence of underlying adenocarcinoma of the colon in patients with acute diverticulitis is ~2% [73].

Stoma Marking

Preoperative ostomy marking by a Wound Care Ostomy (WOC) nurse is generally considered beneficial. Several studies examined preoperative ostomy teaching and marking and concluded teaching improved the quality of life and also reduced postoperative complications [74, 75]. However, additional studies are need to definitively address this question [76]. The ASCRS guidelines for creation and reversal of ostomies are reviewed separately [77].

Preoperative Antibiotics

Antibiotics are indicated for patients undergoing elective, urgent, and emergent surgery for diverticulitis. Several clinical trials studied the roles of oral antibiotics, systemic antibiotics, and mechanical bowel preparations for patients undergoing colectomies. Mechanical bowel preparation by itself does not reduce the incidence of colorectal surgical site infections (SSIs) [69, 70]. In contrast, meta-analysis of several clinical trials showed the combination of oral non-absorbable antibiotics and systemic antibiotics having superior results compared to each regimen used alone [71]. Additional clinical trials are necessary to define the best combination of mechanical bowel preparation and oral/systemic antibiotic regimen for elective colon surgery.

Intraoperative Considerations

Operative Approach (Open versus Laparoscopic versus Robotic)

A modified lithotomy position is recommended to allow intraoperative endoscopic evaluation. The laparoscopic approach is preferred for elective colectomy if expertise is available [42]. Review of 25 randomized clinical trials showed superior short term and equivalent long term outcomes for the laparoscopic approach [78]. Another meta-analysis comparing both approaches revealed significant increases in complications including wound infection, blood transfusion, postoperative ileus, and incisional hernia with the open procedure. Analysis of the National Inpatient Sample confirmed these findings, concluding the laparoscopic operation was associated with lower morbidity, lower mortality, shorter hospital stay, and lower hospital charges compared to an open operation for diverticulitis [79]. The most recent systematic review confirmed these findings and recommendations [80]. Colectomy can be performed using a modified laparoscopic technique, termed single-incision laparoscopic colectomy (SILC), which was shown to be safe and effective [81]. A case control study compared this technique to the traditional multi-port technique and reported overall similar outcomes with better pain scores for patients in the SILC group [82]. Robotic-assisted colectomy has become popular and found to be similar to the laparoscopic approach with respect to length of hospital stay, morbidity, anastomotic leak, and ileus [83]. However, the learning curve is steep for these approaches and more studies are required before nationwide implementation.

Margins of Resection

Surgical procedures for diverticulitis including sigmoidectomy are well described [84]. Several principles of surgical resection are important. Briefly, the abdominal cavity is entered via a midline laparotomy incision (open approach) or multiple port sites (laparoscopic approach). The sigmoid colon is mobilized proximally and distally using either a medial-to-lateral approach or a lateral-to-medial approach, per the surgeon's preference. The proximal resection margin should extend to the soft pliable bowel. The distal resection margin is the proximal rectum where the teniae coli splay out. Recurrence was four times higher in patients with colo-sigmoid anastomosis compared to those with colorectal anastomosis [85]. The splenic flexure should be mobilized, if needed, to perform a tension free anastomosis. In elective/urgent operations, the colorectal anastomosis is performed using an end-to-end anastomosis (EEA) stapler or the hand-sewn technique. In emergent operations, the same steps are followed and dissection is performed in a proximal to distal fashion down to the sacral promontory. The rectal stump is stapled/sewn, and a proximal diverting end colostomy is created.

Leak Testing

Anastomotic leak testing has been shown to minimize clinical leaks. Several studies showed that a positive intraoperative leak test was associated with a significantly increased clinical leak postoperatively. Additionally, there was no difference in clinical leak following hand sewn or stapled anastomoses [86, 87]. In one study, patients with a positive intraoperative anastomotic leak, who underwent anastomotic revision with or without a diverting proximal colostomy, had no clinical leaks. In contrast, 12% of patients who underwent simple suture repair of a leaky anastomosis had a clinical leak [86].

Use of Ureteral Stents

Ureteral injury from colectomy occurs in less than 1% of all cases. Use of ureteral stents, while it may detect injury, was not shown to prevent it. Additionally, the use of stents increases operative times, costs, and adds stent-related complications. This procedure has been discouraged except for complicated cases including those with abnormal anatomy, morbidly obese, and those who had irradiation or reoperation.

Sparing the Superior Hemorrhoidal Artery

Preserving the inferior mesenteric artery (IMA) has been a controversial question for the operating surgeon. Theoretically, preserving the artery could decrease colorectal anastomotic complications but the available results have been mixed. A retrospective review showed no difference [88], but a randomized controlled trial showed a significantly decreased leak when the IMA was left intact [89]. A recent meta-analysis investigated the effect of high verse low ligation of the IMA and demonstrated increased morbidity and leakage with high ligation [90]. While this data suggests low ligation is associated with better outcomes, especially in the absences of neoplastic findings, more data is needed to reach the final conclusion on this question.

Postoperative Considerations

Fast Track Recovery Protocols

The enhanced recovery after surgery (ERAS) is a fast track recovery protocol that has been shown to improve outcomes of elective open and laparoscopic colon surgery for diverticular disease. A meta-analysis of several randomized controlled trials showed decreased length of stay, decreased 30-day morbidity, and similar readmission rate for patients on enhanced recovery protocols compared to patients undergoing traditional care [91]. A single center retrospective study showed a shorter time from surgery to first solid meal (2.3 versus 3.6 days), earlier return of bowel function (2.6 versus 3.5 days), earlier hospital discharge (3 versus 5 days), and fewer complications (15% vs 26%), compared with the control group [92].

Postoperative Complications

The majority of patients report complete recovery after surgical intervention for diverticulitis. However, up to 27 percent continue to complain of persistent abdominal pain in the same location as their prior diverticular disease, prompting further evaluation by gastroenterologists and consideration of other intestinal disorders [93]. Up to 7% of patients continued to report recurrent diverticulitis symptoms, and the majority of these patients were found to have incomplete sigmoid resection rather than development of more proximal diverticular disease [64].

A multi-center prospective clinical trial showed significantly higher mortality, surgical, and medical complication rates for Hartmann's procedure or primary resection with anastomosis. Logistic regression analysis showed the odds of mortality increased based on the Hinchey class from 0.54 (class I), up to 6.18 (class IV). The odds of mortality were 7.48 for urgent procedures and 10.1 for emergent procedures [94]. Other complications of colectomies including ureteral injury, splenic injury, intra-abdominal abscess, enteric fistula, bleeding, and postoperative bowel obstruction have been reviewed extensively [95].

Conclusion

Acute diverticulitis remains a surgical disease. Surgical management continues to evolve as understanding of the pathophysiology of the disease gains more breadth and depth. The outcome of surgical intervention is optimized on several levels. First, encouraging a healthy life style and a balanced high fiber diet is incumbent upon all care providers. Non-operative management should be initiated and optimized to ideally convert an emergent or urgent surgical intervention to an elective operation, thereby minimizing the associated morbidity and mortality. The less invasive surgical approaches and best technical practices should be adopted for the same purpose. An individualized approach to each patient should balance controlling the disease process, restoring physiologic function, and maximize the quality of life. Insight derived from scientific investigation into the microbiome of the gut and well-controlled clinical studies are needed to enhance our management of this disease.

REFERENCES

[1] Etzioni, DA; Mack, TM; Beart, RW; Jr. Kaiser, AM. Diverticulitis in the United States: 1998-2005: changing patterns of disease and treatment. *Ann Surg.*, 2009, 249(2), 210-217.

[2] Teetor, T; Palachick, B; Grim, R; et al. The changing epidemiology of diverticulitis in the United States. *Am Surg.*, 2017, 83(4), e134-136.

[3] Dharmarajan, S; Hunt, SR; Birnbaum, EH; Fleshman, JW; Mutch, MG. The efficacy of nonoperative management of acute complicated diverticulitis. *Dis Colon Rectum.*, 2011, 54(6), 663-671.

[4] Rafferty, J; Shellito, P; Hyman, NH; Buie, WD; Standards Committee of American Society of Colorectal Surgery. Practice parameters for sigmoid diverticulitis. *Dis Colon Rectum.*, 2006, 49(7), 939-944.

[5] Ricciardi, R; Baxter, NN; Read, TE; Marcello, PW; Hall, J; Roberts, PL. Is the decline in the surgical treatment for diverticulitis associated with an increase in complicated diverticulitis? *Dis Colon Rectum.*, 2009, 52(9), 1558-1563.

[6] Kaiser, AM; Jiang, JK; Lake, JP; et al. The management of complicated diverticulitis and the role of computed tomography. *Am J Gastroenterol.*, 2005, 100(4), 910-917.

[7] Ambrosetti, P; Chautems, R; Soravia, C; Peiris-Waser, N; Terrier, F. Long-term outcome of mesocolic and pelvic diverticular abscesses of the left colon: a prospective study of 73 cases. *Dis Colon Rectum.*, 2005, 48(4), 787-791.

[8] Lidsky, ME; Thacker, JK; Lagoo-Deenadayalan, SA; Scarborough, JE. Advanced age is an independent predictor for increased morbidity and mortality after emergent surgery for diverticulitis. *Surgery.*, 2012, 152(3), 465-472.

[9] Vaid, S; Wallet, J; Litt, J; Bell, T; Grim, R; Ahuja, V. Application of a tertiary referral scoring system to predict nonreversal of Hartmann's procedure for diverticulitis in a community hospital. *Am Surg.*, 2011, 77(7), 814-819.

[10] Gervaz, P; Mugnier-Konrad, B; Morel, P; Huber, O; Inan, I. Laparoscopic versus open sigmoid resection for diverticulitis: long-term results of a prospective, randomized trial. *Surg Endosc.* 2011, 25(10), 3373-3378.

[11] Gawlick, U; Nirula, R. Resection and primary anastomosis with proximal diversion instead of Hartmann's: evolving the management of diverticulitis using NSQIP data. *J Trauma Acute Care Surg.*, 2012, 72(4), 807-814, quiz 1124.

[12] Tabbara, M; Velmahos, GC; Butt, MU; et al. Missed opportunities for primary repair in complicated acute diverticulitis. *Surgery.*, 2010, 148(5), 919-924.

[13] White, SI; Frenkiel, B; Martin, PJ. A ten-year audit of perforated sigmoid diverticulitis: highlighting the outcomes of laparoscopic lavage. *Dis Colon Rectum.*, 2010, 53(11), 1537-1541.

[14] Regenbogen, SE; Hardiman, KM; Hendren, S; Morris, AM. Surgery for diverticulitis in the 21st century: a systematic review. *JAMA Surg.*, 2014, 149(3), 292-303.

[15] Peery, AF; Barrett, PR; Park, D; et al. A high-fiber diet does not protect against asymptomatic diverticulosis. *Gastroenterology.*, 2012, 142(2), 266-272 e261.

[16] Cheskin, LJ; Bohlman, M; Schuster, MM. Diverticular disease in the elderly. *Gastroenterol Clin North Am.*, 1990, 19(2), 391-403.

[17] Wong, SK; Ho, YH; Leong, AP; Seow-Choen, F. Clinical behavior of complicated right-sided and left-sided diverticulosis. *Dis Colon Rectum.*, 1997, 40(3), 344-348.

[18] Shahedi, K; Fuller, G; Bolus, R; et al. Long-term risk of acute diverticulitis among patients with incidental diverticulosis found during colonoscopy. *Clin Gastroenterol Hepatol.*, 2013, 11(12), 1609-1613.

[19] Strate, LL; Modi, R; Cohen, E; Spiegel, BM. Diverticular disease as a chronic illness: evolving epidemiologic and clinical insights. *Am J Gastroenterol.*, 2012, 107(10), 1486-1493.

[20] Stollman, NH; Raskin, JB. Diagnosis and management of diverticular disease of the colon in adults. Ad Hoc Practice Parameters Committee of the American College of Gastroenterology. *Am J Gastroenterol.*, 1999, 94(11), 3110-3121.

[21] Bharucha, AE; Parthasarathy, G; Ditah, I; et al. Temporal trends in the incidence and natural history of diverticulitis: a aopulation-based study. *Am J Gastroenterol.*, 2015, 110(11), 1589-1596.

[22] Rege, RV; Nahrwold, DL. Diverticular disease. *Curr Probl Surg.*, 1989, 26(3), 133-189.

[23] Strate, LL; Liu, YL; Syngal, S; Aldoori, WH; Giovannucci, EL. Nut, corn, and popcorn consumption and the incidence of diverticular disease. *JAMA.*, 2008, 300(8), 907-914.

[24] Daniels, L; Unlu, C; de, Korte, N; et al. Randomized clinical trial of observational versus antibiotic treatment for a first episode of CT-proven uncomplicated acute diverticulitis. *Br J Surg.*, 2017, 104(1), 52-61.

[25] Chabok, A; Pahlman, L; Hjern, F; Haapaniemi, S; Smedh, K; Group, AS. Randomized clinical trial of antibiotics in acute uncomplicated diverticulitis. *Br J Surg.*, 2012, 99(4), 532-539.

[26] Humes, DJ; Spiller, RC. Review article: The pathogenesis and management of acute colonic diverticulitis. *Aliment Pharmacol Ther.*, 2014, 39(4), 359-370.

[27] Cao, Y; Strate, LL; Keeley, BR; et al. Meat intake and risk of diverticulitis among men. *Gut.*, 2018, 67(3), 466-472.

[28] Hjern, F; Wolk, A; Hakansson, N. Obesity, physical inactivity, and colonic diverticular disease requiring hospitalization in women: a prospective cohort study. *Am J Gastroenterol.*, 2012, 107(2), 296-302.

[29] Kvasnovsky, CL; Papagrigoriadis, S; Bjarnason, I. Increased diverticular complications with nonsteriodal anti-inflammatory drugs and other medications: a systematic review and meta-analysis. *Colorectal Dis.*, 2014, 16(6), O189-196.

[30] Hjern, F; Wolk, A; Hakansson, N. Smoking and the risk of diverticular disease in women. *Br J Surg.*, 2011, 98(7), 997-1002.

[31] Aune, D; Sen, A; Leitzmann, MF; Tonstad, S; Norat, T; Vatten, LJ. Tobacco smoking and the risk of diverticular disease - a systematic review and meta-analysis of prospective studies. *Colorectal Dis.*, 2017, 19(7), 621-633.

[32] Strate, LL; Liu, YL; Aldoori, WH; Giovannucci, EL. Physical activity decreases diverticular complications. *Am J Gastroenterol.*, 2009, 104(5), 1221-1230.

[33] Liu, PH; Cao, Y; Keeley, BR; et al. Adherence to a healthy lifestyle is associated with a lower risk of diverticulitis among men. *Am J Gastroenterol.*, 2017, 112(12), 1868-1876.

[34] Wheat, CL; Strate LL. Trends in Hospitalization for Diverticulitis and Diverticular Bleeding in the United States From 2000 to 2010. *Clin Gastroenterol Hepatol.*, 2016, 14(1), 96-103 e101.

[35] Sugihara, K; Muto, T; Morioka, Y; Asano, A; Yamamoto, T. Diverticular disease of the colon in Japan. A review of 615 cases. *Dis Colon Rectum.*, 1984, 27(8), 531-537.

[36] Maguire, LH; Song, M; Strate, LL; Giovannucci, EL; Chan, AT. Association of geographic and seasonal variation with diverticulitis admissions. *JAMA Surg.*, 2015, 150(1), 74-77.

[37] Nikberg, M; Ji, J; Leppert, J; Sundquist, K; Chabok, A. Socioeconomic characteristics and comorbidities of diverticular disease in Sweden 1997-2012. *Int J Colorectal Dis.*, 2017, 32(11), 1591-1596.

[38] Hjern, F; Johansson, C; Mellgren, A; Baxter, NN; Hjern, A. Diverticular disease and migration--the influence of acculturation to a Western lifestyle on diverticular disease. *Aliment Pharmacol Ther.*, 2006, 23(6), 797-805.

[39] Young-Fadok, TM. Diverticulitis. *N Engl J Med.*, 2019, 380(5), 500-501.

[40] Jacobs, DO. Clinical practice. Diverticulitis. *N Engl J Med.*, 2007, 357(20), 2057-2066.

[41] Andeweg, CS; Wegdam, JA; Groenewoud, J; van der, Wilt, GJ; van Goor, H; Bleichrodt, RP. Toward an evidence-based step-up approach in diagnosing diverticulitis. *Scand J Gastroenterol.*, 2014, 49(7), 775-784.

[42] Feingold, D; Steele, SR; Lee, S; et al. Practice parameters for the treatment of sigmoid diverticulitis. *Dis Colon Rectum.*, 2014, 57(3), 284-294.

[43] Sarma, D; Longo, WE; NDSG. Diagnostic imaging for diverticulitis. *J Clin Gastroenterol.*, 2008, 42(10), 1139-1141.

[44] McKee, RF; Deignan, RW; Krukowski, ZH. Radiological investigation in acute diverticulitis. *Br J Surg.*, 1993, 80(5), 560-565.

[45] Hinchey, EJ; Schaal, PG; Richards, GK. Treatment of perforated diverticular disease of the colon. *Adv Surg.*, 1978, 12, 85-109.

[46] Klarenbeek, BR; de Korte, N; van der Peet, DL; Cuesta, MA. Review of current classifications for diverticular disease and a translation into clinical practice. *Int J Colorectal Dis.*, 2012, 27(2), 207-214.

[47] Biondo, S; Golda, T; Kreisler, E; et al. Outpatient versus hospitalization management for uncomplicated diverticulitis: a prospective, multicenter randomized clinical trial (DIVER Trial). *Ann Surg.*, 2014, 259(1), 38-44.

[48] Stollman, N; Smalley, W; Hirano, I; Committee, AGAICG. American Gastroenterological Association Institute Guideline on the Management of Acute Diverticulitis. *Gastroenterology.*, 2015, 149(7), 1944-1949.

[49] Broderick-Villa, G; Burchette, RJ; Collins, JC; Abbas, MA; Haigh, PI. Hospitalization for acute diverticulitis does not mandate routine elective colectomy. *Arch Surg.*, 2005, 140(6), 576-581, discussion 581-573.

[50] Guzzo, J; Hyman, N. Diverticulitis in young patients: is resection after a single attack always warranted? *Dis Colon Rectum.*, 2004, 47(7), 1187-1190, discussion 1190-1181.

[51] Hjern, F; Josephson, T; Altman, D; Holmstrom, B; Johansson, C. Outcome of younger patients with acute diverticulitis. *Br J Surg.*, 2008, 95(6), 758-764.

[52] Lidor, AO; Schneider, E; Segal, J; Yu, Q; Feinberg, R; Wu, AW. Elective surgery for diverticulitis is associated with high risk of intestinal diversion and hospital readmission in older adults. *J Gastrointest Surg.*, 2010, 14(12), 1867-1873, discussion 1873-1864.

[53] Egger, B; Peter, MK; Candinas, D. Persistent symptoms after elective sigmoid resection for diverticulitis. *Dis Colon Rectum.*, 2008, 51(7), 1044-1048.

[54] Levack, MM; Savitt, LR; Berger, DL; et al. Sigmoidectomy syndrome? Patients' perspectives on the functional outcomes following surgery for diverticulitis. *Dis Colon Rectum.*, 2012, 55(1), 10-17.

[55] Andeweg, C; Peters, J; Bleichrodt, R; van Goor, H. Incidence and risk factors of recurrence after surgery for pathology-proven diverticular disease. *World J Surg.*, 2008, 32(7), 1501-1506.

[56] van de Wall, BJM; Stam, MAW; Draaisma, WA; et al. Surgery versus conservative management for recurrent and ongoing left-sided diverticulitis (DIRECT trial): an open-label, multicentre, randomised controlled trial. *Lancet Gastroenterol Hepatol.*, 2017, 2(1), 13-22.

[57] Altman, D; Forsgren, C; Hjern, F; Lundholm, C; Cnattingius, S; Johansson, AL. Influence of hysterectomy on fistula formation in women with diverticulitis. *Br J Surg.*, 2010, 97(2), 251-257.

[58] Hwang, SS; Cannom, RR; Abbas, MA; Etzioni, D. Diverticulitis in transplant patients and patients on chronic corticosteroid therapy: a systematic review. *Dis Colon Rectum.*, 2010, 53(12), 1699-1707.

[59] Klarenbeek, BR; Samuels, M; van der Wal, MA; van der Peet, DL; Meijerink, WJ; Cuesta, MA. Indications for elective sigmoid resection in diverticular disease. *Ann Surg.*, 2010, 251(4), 670-674.

[60] Siewert, B; Tye, G; Kruskal, J; et al. Impact of CT-guided drainage in the treatment of diverticular abscesses: size matters. *AJR Am J Roentgenol.*, 2006, 186(3), 680-686.

[61] Kumar, RR; Kim, JT; Haukoos, JS; et al. Factors affecting the successful management of intra-abdominal abscesses with antibiotics and the need for percutaneous drainage. *Dis Colon Rectum.*, 2006, 49(2), 183-189.

[62] Oberkofler, CE; Rickenbacher, A; Raptis, DA; et al. A multicenter randomized clinical trial of primary anastomosis or Hartmann's procedure for perforated left colonic diverticulitis with purulent or fecal peritonitis. *Ann Surg.*, 2012, 256(5), 819-826, discussion 826-817.

[63] Bridoux, V; Regimbeau, JM; Ouaissi, M; et al. Hartmann's procedure or primary anastomosis for generalized peritonitis due to perforated diverticulitis: a prospective multicenter randomized trial (DIVERTI). *J Am Coll Surg.*, 2017, 225(6), 798-805.

[64] Benn, PL; Wolff, BG; Ilstrup, DM. Level of anastomosis and recurrent colonic diverticulitis. *Am J Surg.*, 1986, 151(2), 269-271.

[65] Cirocchi, R; Afshar, S; Di Saverio, S; et al. A historical review of surgery for peritonitis secondary to acute colonic diverticulitis: from Lockhart-Mummery to evidence-based medicine. *World J Emerg Surg.*, 2017, 12, 14.

[66] Stumpf, MJ; Vinces, FY; Edwards, J. Is primary anastomosis safe in the surgical management of complications of acute diverticulitis? *Am Surg.*, 2007, 73(8), 787-790, discussion 790-781.

[67] Balanzoni, S; Perrucci, A; Pasi, L; Montanari, MC. [The Hartmann intervention. The current indications and the authors' own experience]. *Minerva Chir.*, 1997, 52(4), 383-386.

[68] Strate, LL; Morris, AM. Epidemiology, Pathophysiology, and Treatment of Diverticulitis. *Gastroenterology.*, 2019. Is this a book chapter?)

[69] Fry, DE. Colon preparation and surgical site infection. *Am J Surg.*, 2011, 202(2), 225-232.

[70] Guenaga, KF; Matos, D; Wille-Jorgensen, P. Mechanical bowel preparation for elective colorectal surgery. *Cochrane Database Syst Rev.*, 2011(9), CD001544.

[71] McSorley, ST; Steele, CW; McMahon, AJ. Meta-analysis of oral antibiotics, in combination with preoperative intravenous antibiotics and mechanical bowel preparation the day before surgery, compared with intravenous antibiotics and mechanical bowel preparation alone

to reduce surgical-site infections in elective colorectal surgery. *BJS Open.*, 2018, 2(4), 185-194.

[72] Wolff, JH; Rubin, A; Potter, JD; et al. Clinical significance of colonoscopic findings associated with colonic thickening on computed tomography: is colonoscopy warranted when thickening is detected? *J Clin Gastroenterol.*, 2008, 42(5), 472-475.

[73] Sai, VF; Velayos, F; Neuhaus, J; Westphalen, AC. Colonoscopy after CT diagnosis of diverticulitis to exclude colon cancer: a systematic literature review. *Radiology.*, 2012, 263(2), 383-390.

[74] Gulbiniene, J; Markelis, R; Tamelis, A; Saladzinskas, Z. [The impact of preoperative stoma siting and stoma care education on patient's quality of life]. *Medicina (Kaunas).*, 2004, 40(11), 1045-1053.

[75] Bass, EM; Del Pino, A; Tan, A; Pearl, RK; Orsay, CP; Abcarian, H. Does preoperative stoma marking and education by the enterostomal therapist affect outcome? *Dis Colon Rectum.*, 1997, 40(4), 440-442.

[76] Colwell, JC; Gray, M. Does preoperative teaching and stoma site marking affect surgical outcomes in patients undergoing ostomy surgery? *J Wound Ostomy Continence Nurs.*, 2007, 34(5), 492-496.

[77] Hendren, S; Hammond, K; Glasgow, SC; et al. Clinical practice guidelines for ostomy surgery. *Dis Colon Rectum.*, 2015, 58(4), 375-387.

[78] Schwenk, W; Haase, O; Neudecker, J; Muller, JM. Short term benefits for laparoscopic colorectal resection. *Cochrane Database Syst Rev.*, 2005(3), CD003145.

[79] Masoomi, H; Buchberg, B; Nguyen, B; Tung, V; Stamos, MJ; Mills, S. Outcomes of laparoscopic versus open colectomy in elective surgery for diverticulitis. *World J Surg.*, 2011, 35(9), 2143-2148.

[80] Wu, KL; Lee, KC; Liu, CC; Chen, HH; Lu, CC. Laparoscopic versus open surgery for diverticulitis: a systematic review and meta-analysis. *Dig Surg.*, 2017, 34(3), 203-215.

[81] Vestweber, B; Galetin, T; Lammerting, K; et al. Single-incision laparoscopic surgery: outcomes from 224 colonic resections performed at a single center using SILS. *Surg Endosc.*, 2013, 27(2), 434-442.

[82] Champagne, BJ; Papaconstantinou, HT; Parmar, SS; et al. Single-incision versus standard multiport laparoscopic colectomy: a multicenter, case-controlled comparison. *Ann Surg.*, 2012, 255(1), 66-69.

[83] Ragupathi, M; Ramos-Valadez, DI; Patel, CB; Haas, EM. Robotic-assisted laparoscopic surgery for recurrent diverticulitis: experience in consecutive cases and a review of the literature. *Surg Endosc.*, 2011, 25(1), 199-206.

[84] Zollinger, RM. The atlas of surgical operations: Elliott Carr Cutler and Robert Zollinger. *American Journal of Surgery.*, 2003, 186(3), 211-216.

[85] Thaler, K; Baig, MK; Berho, M; et al. Determinants of recurrence after sigmoid resection for uncomplicated diverticulitis. *Dis Colon Rectum.*, 2003, 46(3), 385-388.

[86] Ricciardi, R; Roberts, PL; Marcello, PW; Hall, JF; Read, TE; Schoetz, DJ. Anastomotic leak testing after colorectal resection: what are the data? *Arch Surg.*, 2009, 144(5), 407-411, discussion 411-402.

[87] Beard, JD; Nicholson, ML; Sayers, RD; Lloyd, D; Everson, NW. Intraoperative air testing of colorectal anastomoses: a prospective, randomized trial. *Br J Surg.*, 1990, 77(10), 1095-1097.

[88] Lehmann, RK; Brounts, LR; Johnson, EK; Rizzo, JA; Steele, SR. Does sacrifice of the inferior mesenteric artery or superior rectal artery affect anastomotic leak following sigmoidectomy for diverticulitis? A retrospective review. *Am J Surg.*, 2011, 201(5), 623-627.

[89] Tocchi, A; Mazzoni, G; Fornasari, V; Miccini, M; Daddi, G; Tagliacozzo, S. Preservation of the inferior mesenteric artery in colorectal resection for complicated diverticular disease. *Am J Surg.*, 2001, 182(2), 162-167.

[90] Zeng, J; Su, G. High ligation of the inferior mesenteric artery during sigmoid colon and rectal cancer surgery increases the risk of anastomotic leakage: a meta-analysis. *World J Surg Oncol.*, 2018, 16(1), 157.

[91] Adamina, M; Kehlet, H; Tomlinson, GA; Senagore, AJ; Delaney, CP. Enhanced recovery pathways optimize health outcomes and resource

utilization: a meta-analysis of randomized controlled trials in colorectal surgery. *Surgery.*, 2011, 149(6), 830-840.

[92] Larson, DW; Batdorf, NJ; Touzios, JG; et al. A fast-track recovery protocol improves outcomes in elective laparoscopic colectomy for diverticulitis. *J Am Coll Surg.*, 2010, 211(4), 485-489.

[93] Wolff, BG; Ready, RL; MacCarty, RL; Dozois, RR; Beart, RW. Jr. Influence of sigmoid resection on progression of diverticular disease of the colon. *Dis Colon Rectum.*, 1984, 27(10), 645-647.

[94] Constantinides, VA; Tekkis, PP; Senapati, A; Association of Coloproctology of Great Britain, I. Prospective multicentre evaluation of adverse outcomes following treatment for complicated diverticular disease. *Br J Surg.*, 2006, 93(12), 1503-1513.

[95] Longo, WE; Virgo, KS; Johnson, FE; et al. Risk factors for morbidity and mortality after colectomy for colon cancer. *Dis Colon Rectum.*, 2000, 43(1), 83-91.

In: Diverticulitis: Diagnosis and Treatment ISBN: 978-1-53618-081-7
Editors: Shams-ul-Bari et al.

Chapter 5

MANAGEMENT OF ACUTE DIVERTICULITIS IN IMMUNODEFFICIENT PATIENTS

Laura Colao García[1,*]***, Javier Serrano González***[2] ***and Jesús Gabriel García Schiever***[3]
Laura Colao García; Surgery Department of University Hospital of Torrejón de Ardoz, Madrid, Spain
Javier Serrano González, Surgery Department of University Hospital of Torrejón de Ardoz, Madrid, Spain
Jesús Gabriel García Schiever, Surgery Department of Hospital General Universitario de Ciudad Real, Ciudad Real, Spain

ABSTRACT

Management of acute diverticulitis has been changing in the past several years. A conservative treatment of uncomplicated acute diverticulitis is the most common approach. Surgical treatment of the complicated cases was mandatory and unquestionable during the first half of the 20th century. Currently, surgery is the last option in the management

---

* Corresponding Author's E mail: lauracg007@hotmail.com.

of acute diverticulitis and is limited to cases with free perforation, peritonitis and/or sepsis.

Immunodeficiency can mask the clinical manifestations of the disease, and may alter capacity of the patient to defend itself from the local or generalized infection due to acute diverticulitis. Patients with immunodeficiency have a higher risk of conservative treatment failure. They also have a greater chance of complication in their first episode of acute diverticulitis, such as free perforation; these complications are also likely to be more severe than in immunocompetent patients. Immunodeficiency seems to have a great impact on the morbidity and mortality of these patients. This impact is such that a proposal for elective sigmoidectomy in patients with previous episodes of acute diverticulitis and in patients who are on a wait list for transplant surgery has been made. This strategy would aim to prevent the patient's death. The last two decades have witnessed constant change in the diagnosis and treatment of acute diverticulitis in immunocompromised patients, even more than in immunocompetent patients. There are strong controversies regarding treatment and management timeline.

With the available information, no strict recommendations can be made for the management of acute diverticulitis in immunocompromised patients. Treatment of the first episode of acute diverticulitis in this group of patients is similar to immunocompetent patients. Prophylactic elective surgery can be recommended in selected patients with a higher risk of developing further episodes of complicated acute diverticulitis. Some of these patients include those on immunosuppression treatment, chronic kidney disease, collagen vascular disease, patients on a wait list for transplant or with autosomal dominant polycystic disease.

INTRODUCTION

The incidence of colonic diverticular disease is rising in developed countries, and its prevalence increases with age. Mean age of the population and the proportion of the elderly people involved in developed countries is increasing; consequently, diverticular disease is a growing problem and diagnostic and treatment strategies for management of this disease should be established.

Prevalence of diverticulosis in different age groups and different genders can be summarized as follows [1].

- Prevalence as per the age groups;
  - <40 years: 5%
  - 40-60 years: 30%
  - 60-80 years: 65%
- Prevalence according to gender;
  - <50 years: More frequent in males
  - 50–70 years: Slightly more frequent in females
  - 70 years: More frequent in females

Diverticula can be defined as small out-pouches in the intestinal wall, usually asymptomatic. When symptoms develop, these can include hemorrhage, acute diverticulitis and segmental colitis. Diverticulitis occurs when a diverticulum becomes inflamed. These diverticula are usually false diverticula or pseudodiverticula. In these the mucosa and submucosa protrude through the muscle layer and are covered only by the serosa. They usually appear at weak points where the vasa recta penetrate the muscle layer of the colonic wall to irrigate the mucosa and submucosa.

The development of colonic diverticulosis is multifactorial. Its etiology has been widely studied, diet being the most studied cause. A low fiber diet with absence of soluble fiber in the colon increases the intraluminal pressure during colonic peristalsis. Soluble fiber increases the volume of fecal matter. This increase in the intraluminal pressure leads to formation of out pouches and diverticulae formation. [2]. A red meat enriched diet, obesity, sedentary lifestyle and smoking are independent factors that increase the risk for acute diverticulitis [3]. It has classically been considered that seeds, nuts, and popcorn are not associated with an increased risk of diverticulosis and diverticular disease, nor are caffeine and alcohol [4]. Smoking, on the other hand, is not only associated with diverticular disease, but also appears to increase the risk of perforation and abscess formation [5]. Certain drugs also play a significant role in the pathogenesis of the diverticular disease. While non-steroidal anti-inflammatory drugs, steroids, and opiates are associated with an increased risk for diverticulitis and diverticular hemorrhage, vitamin D and statins bestow a protective effect [5, 6, 7].

Diverticulae are usually located in the sigmoid colon. However, in Asian countries they are located mainly in the right colon. Colonic diverticulosis affects up to 10% of the population. The elderly, as we have mentioned before, are more vulnerable to this condition. As a matter of fact, 50% of the population over 50 years of age have diverticulosis, with a higher prevalence in the female population. Less than 5% of the population have it before the age of 40 years and most of them are obese males [1].

It has been traditionally considered that 15-25% of patients with diverticulosis would develop acute diverticulitis during their lifetime [8, 9]. However, this data is based on colon cancer screening studies, after performing a colonoscopy. These studies tend to underestimate the real prevalence of diverticulosis in the general population. More recent studies suggest that the incidence of acute diverticulitis is <5% [10, 11]. Younger patients have a higher incidence of acute diverticulitis per year of life than the older population. This raises doubts about the traditional perception of how often diverticulosis progresses into acute diverticulitis [8, 9, 12-15].

Acute diverticulitis is the most common complication of the diverticular disease. It occurs when there is an erosion of its mucosa, probably due to fecoliths, and this ulcer degenerates into a necrotizing inflammation of the diverticulum [16]. Rectal bleeding develops in 3-5% of patients with diverticulosis, and up to 40% of cases of lower gastrointestinal hemorrhages are secondary to diverticulosis [17]. Since the most common location of diverticulosis is the sigmoid colon, the most frequent clinical presentation of acute diverticulitis is pain in the left iliac fossa. This pain can radiate to the hypogastrium, or even to the right iliac fossa in cases of a redundant sigmoid colon.

Diagnosis is based on the clinical presentation of the patients, like pain in the left iliac fossa and hypogastrium, fever, dysuria, tenesmus, with or without rectal bleeding or other pathological substances in feces, constipation or diarrhea. Laboratory tests show results compatible with an infection, such as a high white cell count and neutrophilia, as well as other inflammatory indicators, such as a high reactive C protein. In any case, definitive diagnosis must include radiologic imaging. CT has shown the highest sensitivity and specificity for diagnosing this disease with a sensitivity of around 94%, and specificity 99%. This imaging test can also assess the degree of the disease, as well as the presence of possible complications.

The severity of the disease can be classified on the basis of Modified Hinchey Classification [18,19] into the following stages.

Stage 0: Mild clinical diverticulitis
Stage Ia: Confined pericolic inflammation, no abscess
Stage Ib: Confined pericolic inflammation, abscess of less than 2 cm
Stage II: Pelvic, retroperitoneal or distant abscess greater than 2 cm
Stage III: Generalized purulent peritonitis, no communication with colonic lumen
Stage IV: Fecal peritonitis, open communication with colonic lumen

In order to avoid the radiation exposure associated with CT, a high resolution abdomino-pelvic ultrasound can be performed. Its sensitivity and specificity are similar to the CT, although it is operator dependent. It also has the limitation of making it more difficult to compare further studies during the evolution of a patient. Colonoscopy should not be performed during an episode of acute diverticulitis, given the high risk of injury or perforation of the colonic wall.

Management of acute diverticulitis has been changing in the past several years. Surgical treatment of the complicated cases was mandatory and unquestionable during the first half of the 20th century; currently, surgery is the last option in the management of acute diverticulitis and is limited to cases with free perforation, peritonitis and/or sepsis.

A conservative treatment of uncomplicated acute diverticulitis is the most common approach. This mainly consists of a relative rest to the digestive tract and in some cases, this measure alone could be enough. Oral antibiotics can be added in those cases which are associated with risk factors. Admission and intravenous antibiotics may be required in cases with low degree complicated acute diverticulitis with or without risk factors.

If the patient also presents a pericolic or intramesenteric abscess of less than 5 cm in diameter, a conservative management could still be appropriate, using intravenous antibiotics along with rest to the digestive tract. If the abscess is greater than 5 cm, radiology guided percutaneous drainage should be considered, and performed if there is a wide enough window to do so.

When surgery is considered, due to complications such as free perforation, severe sepsis or peritonitis, several options are available. The best option should be chosen considering the patient's comorbidities, the severity of the acute episode and the surgeon's expertise. These different options include laparoscopic lavage and drainage, segmental colonic resection with or without primary anastomosis, and with or without ileostomy. Segmental colonic resection with terminal colostomy has been classically considered the safest treatment for most surgeons, in spite of the fact that further reconstructive surgery is not free of morbidity and mortality.

Acute Diverticulitis in Immunodefficient Patients

The concept of diverticular disease has been explained, including a brief description of its incidence, prevalence, pathogenesis, evolution, diagnosis and the most common treatment options. The issue which will be addressed is the management of this condition in immunocompromised patients.

Multiple studies and publications can be found in medical literature analyzing the process of diverticular disease in *immunocompromised* patients. These patients include:

- Patients on chronic *corticoid* therapies, and on immunosuppressive therapy for various diseases such as myasthenia gravis, Sjögren syndrome, COPD, rheumatoid arthritis, sarcoidosis, ankylosing spondylitis, adrenal insufficiency or psoriasis.
- Patients on immunosuppressive therapy after a solid organ transplant.
- Patients with a malignant extra-colonic neoplasm, including synchronic hematologic diseases with the first episode of acute diverticulitis.
- Patients with chronic kidney disease, stages III to V.

- Patients on other immunosuppressive therapies, such as azathioprine, cyclosporine, methotrexate, tacrolimus, biologic drugs, etc. These drugs are usually used to treat certain diseases, like rheumatoid arthritis, inflammatory bowel disease, myasthenia gravis, Wegener's granulomatosis and hypoderma gangrenosum.

This immunosuppressed condition must be known at least 2 months prior to the first episode of acute diverticulitis. Chronic corticoid treatment is considered when the patient takes at least 5 or 10 mg of methylprednisolone or an equivalent steroidal drug for at least 3 months, and there is a need to continue this treatment [20].

In studies between 2005 and 2010, immunodeficiency was defined as regular treatment with corticoid drugs for a medical reason, either orally or intravenously, for at least 30 days before the current acute episode. Short treatment cycles were not included. Topical, inhaled or rectal treatments were not considered as chronic corticoid treatments [21].

Other diseases that can be included in this group are emphysema, pulmonary fibrosis, AIDS and collagen vascular disease [12].

PREVALENCE

Different studies have observed that immunocompromised patients have a higher tendency or predisposition to develop acute diverticulitis when compared with the immunocompetent population (1% vs 0.02%) [9, 20, 22, 27]. A systematic review on acute diverticulitis in patients after a transplant or with chronic corticoid treatment has described an incidence of 0.4% to 9%. The average incidence was 1%, as aforementioned. Among these patients, those with known diverticulosis have an incidence of diverticular disease of up to 16%, with an average incidence of 8%.

This review also describes that in the study performed by Sawyer et al, transplant patients with or without renal polycystic disease had an incidence of 57% for acute diverticulitis. The study from McCune et al. describes an incidence of 0%. In those patients that had a confirmed absence of diverticulosis before the transplant, neither study reported cases of acute diverticulitis [9, 27,28].

Clinical Manifestations

- Acute diverticulitis in immunodefficient patients has been associated with a worse evolution. This is probably due to a delayed diagnosis and a greater difficulty for these patients to confront infectious diseases. These patients have a more latent clinical manifestation, and not as specific. 92% patients present with abdominal pain, 65% have a high white cell count, 63% have abdominal tenderness, 56% have fever and 50% have hypotension [29-39].

Diagnosis

There are no differences when compared to the general population. Although, given that their clinical manifestations are less intense and typical, a higher degree of suspicion is needed to successfully reach to a diagnosis.

Evolution

The evolution of the disease in these immunocompromised patients has also been described, both in the acute episodes and its recurrences. The guidelines of the America Society of Colon and Rectal Surgeons (ASCRS) for the management of acute diverticulitis describe the fact that immunocompromised patients have a higher failure rate with a conservative management. It also points out that they have a higher mortality rate as well [8, 9]. Studies also describe a higher need for emergency surgical treatment (40% vs 10-25%), as well as a higher mortality rate after emergency surgery (30% vs 5%), when compared to immunocompetent patients [9, 20, 22-26].

In a study from Andreas Brandl et al. [40], 227 patients were recruited between 2008 and 2014, out of which 15 were immunocompromised patients. The latter showed a higher rate of complicated acute diverticulitis (Hinchey ≥ 2, $p = 0.039$) and a higher emergency surgery rate (66.7% vs 29.2%, $p = 0.004$). They also had a longer stay in an Intensive Care Unit (9.8 ± 16.4 days vs 1.2 ± 4.2 days, $p < 0.001$) and more days of admission (27.6 ± 23.5 days vs 14.5 ± 19.9 days, $p = 0.016$). When comparing complications during their admission, immunocompromised patients had more pulmonary complications (33.3% vs 4.7%, $p < 0.001$) and kidney failure (13.3% vs 1.4%, $p = 0.002$); other complications showed no statistically significant differences, such as urinary tract infection ($p = 0.55$), surgical infection ($p = 0.11$), cardiovascular complications ($p = 0.05$), gastrointestinal complications ($p = 0.22$), allergies ($p = 0.71$) and neurological complications ($p = 0.64$). Risk factors associated with hospital mortality were age ($p = 0.008$), perforated acute diverticulitis with generalized peritonitis ($p = 0.007$), the need for emergency surgery ($p = 0.001$), a reactive C protein >20mg/dl ($p = 0.049$) and immunodeficiency ($p = 0.049$). After a linear regression analysis, age (OR 2.57, $p = 0.008$) and emergency surgery (OR 3.03, $p = 0.003$) were identified as significant parameters [40].

Biondo, et al. [20] recruited 1181 patients between 1994 and 2013. Out of these patients, 192 were immunocompromised. This study describes how male gender ($p = 0.012$) and severity of the diverticulitis ($p < 0.001$) have a statistically significant relationship with a higher rate of emergency surgery during the first episode of acute diverticulitis. A multivariate analysis showed that only age and the ASA scale have an association with perioperative mortality. This mortality rate proved to be higher in this study in immunocompromised patients than in the general population (30.7%). From the analysis, the only variable related with a higher surgery rate during the hospital admission was chronic corticoid treatment. Corticoids can mask the clinical manifestations of the disease and of sepsis, which delays a proper diagnosis, and that would explain its relation with the higher surgery rate [20].

The study from Samdani Tushar et al. [41] included 131 patients from 1988 to 2004 who had received chemotherapy during the month prior to the episode of acute diverticulitis. This study compared these patients with those who had not received this type of treatment during the mentioned period of time. In this study, there was no statistically significant differences between the severity of the disease between two groups of patients (13.2% vs 4.4%, $p = 0.12$). Chemotherapy was resumed after an average of 2 months. There were no differences in failure of conservative treatment (13.2% vs 4.4%, $p = 0.12$) and recurrences rate (20.5% vs 18.5%). However, patients with chemotherapy had a higher chance of need of emergency surgery (75% vs 23.5&, $p = 0.03$) and of developing postoperative complications (100% vs 9.1%, $p < 0.01$). Global mortality was also greater among patients who had received chemotherapy [41].

RECURRENCES

Samdani's study [41] also observed that *recurrences* in patients with previous chemotherapy were more severe (87.5% vs 29.4%, $p = 0.01$), although recurrence was as common as in those patients without previous chemotherapy (20.5% vs 18.5%). There were no significant differences between both groups in cumulative probability. Patients with chemothe-rapy had a higher chance of emergency surgery during a recurrent episode (75% vs 23.5%, $p = 0.03$), and also a higher need of an intestinal stoma during this surgery (100% vs 25%, $p = 0.03$). Global mortality during the recurrent episode was still higher in patients who had received chemotherapy. There seemed to be a tendency to a more rare use of conservative management in patients with previous chemotherapy, but with no statistical significance (50% vs 88.1%, $p = 0.06$). No differences in failure of conservative treatment were observed.

Biondo et al. [12] recruited a total of 931 patients from 1994 to 2008, which included 166 immunocompromised and 765 immunocompetent patients. After excluding all those patients who underwent surgery in their first episode of acute diverticulitis, only 657 patients were left, out of which, 107 were immunocompromised and 550 were immunocompetent patients. Recurrence rates were studied in these patients. Maximum follow-up was of

81.62 months. A total of 136 patients (20.7%) developed one or more episodes of acute diverticulitis (21.5% of the immunocompromised patients and 20.5% of the immunocompetent ones). No statistically significant differences were found between two groups (p = 0.82, RR = 1.05, 95%IC 0.70-1.56). 16.4% had one recurrence, 3% had two and 1.3% had three or more recurrent episodes. No association was found between the severity of the first episode and the recurrence rate or the need for emergency surgery in this same study. Immunocompromised patients with a severe first episode did show a significant higher recurrence rate, as well as more severe recurrent episodes. However, there were no differences with immunocompetent patients regarding need for emergency surgery. Recurrence rates were highest during the first 6 months.

In another study by Klarenbeek et al. [10], 291 patients were recruited between 1990 and 2000. These patients received a conservative or a surgical management. After analyzing the data, they described certain risk factors that were more prevalent among patients who underwent emergency surgery. These patients were five times more likely to have a perforation during a recurrent episode of acute diverticulitis than the rest of the patients from the study (36% vs 7%). These risk factors included immunosuppressive treatment, chronic kidney disease, collagen vascular disease and an anesthetic risk of ASA >II.

TREATMENT

Treatment for acute diverticulitis has changed during the past several years. Surgical treatment was mandatory and uncontested for complicated acute diverticulitis during the first half of the 20th century. However, nowadays, surgical treatment is a last resource during the management of acute diverticulitis and is indicated in patients with a free perforation, peritonitis or sepsis.

A conservative treatment of uncomplicated acute diverticulitis is the most common approach. This mainly consists in a relative digestive rest; in some cases, this measure alone could be enough. Oral antibiotics can be added to the treatment in those cases with associated risk factors, or even admission and intravenous antibiotics in low degree complicated acute diverticulitis with or without risk factors. If there is a pericolic or intramesenteric abscess of less than 5cm, conservative management can still be an option, combining a soft diet and intravenous antibiotics. If the abscess is greater than 5cm and has a wide enough radiologic window, percutaneous drainage is indicated.

When there is a free perforation, severe sepsis or peritonitis, surgical treatment is considered. There are various options to perform, considering the patient's comorbidities, the severity of the acute episode and the surgeon's experience. One option is laparoscopic lavage and drainage; another would be a segmental colonic resection with or without primary anastomosis and with or without a diverting ileostomy. Classically, most surgeons consider segmental resection and terminal colostomy the safest option, although, further reconstructive surgery is not free of its morbidity and mortality.

Different results can be found regarding the management of acute diverticulitis in the immunocompromised patient. Historically, it has been always considered that immunocompromised patients not only had a higher risk of developing acute diverticulitis, but also had more severe episodes and more complex recurrences. This was considered to the point that some authors even recommended surgical treatment for even the first episode of acute diverticulitis, without considering a conservative treatment. Also, elective prophylactic sigmoidectomy has been suggested after the first episode to avoid more severe recurrences [42].

The aforementioned study of Samdani et al. [41] also showed that patients with chemotherapy did not have a higher rate of complicated acute diverticulitis during the first episode as compared to patients who were not on chemotherapy (61.5% vs 47.8%, $p = 0.15$). Failure of a conservative medical management was rare in both groups (13.2% vs 4.4%, $p = 0.12$) and the proportion of patients with an intestinal stoma after emergency surgery was similar in both groups (71.45% vs 79.2%, $p = 0.70$). The incidence of postoperative complications was the same in both groups (50% vs 50%, $p = 0.9$), as well as days of admission and mortality rate. Recurrence had no statistical significant differences between both groups (20.5% vs 18.5%). There was a certain tendency towards a lower proportion of conservative management of the recurrent episodes in patients with previous chemotherapy, but without statistical significance (50% vs 88.1%, $p = 0.06$). Failure of conservative management was similar in both groups. With all of this taken into consideration, sigmoidectomy could not be recommended either during the episode of acute diverticulitis or as an elective prophylactic surgery after the acute episode.

- Studies conducted by Biondo et al. [12, 20] on the evolution of acute diverticulitis describe that, in immunocompromised patients, male gender ($p = 0.012$) and severity of the acute diverticulitis ($p < 0.001$) are associated with a higher risk of emergency surgery during the first episode of acute diverticulitis. They also observed that immunocompromised patients had a higher rate of emergency surgery, but only age ($p = 0.039$) and the ASA scale (<0.001) were associated with a higher postoperative mortality. After a conservative management, there was a recurrence rate of 27.8% with severe episodes in 33%. Recurrences were more frequent during the first year. There was an association between the severity of the first episode and the recurrence rate. (HR 2.85, 95% CI 1.14-7.14). Corticoid treatment as cause for immunosuppression was the only risk factor found to be associated with a higher risk of emergency surgery during the first episode of acute diverticulitis. No association was described with postoperative mortality after emergency surgery, or with recurrence rate after conservative management. They concluded that prophylactic surgery in immunocompromised patients with diverticulosis is controversial, since its usefulness is yet unknown in immunocompetent patients. They also recommended a close follow-up of these patients during the first year, with a high grade of suspicion to detect recurrences or persistent diverticulitis. Need for elective surgery should be assessed individually.

Brandl et al. [40] reported that immunocompromised patients needed more days of admission (27.6 vs 14.5, $p = 0.016$), more days in an ICU (9.8

vs 1.1, $p < 0.001$), had a higher rate of emergency surgery (66% vs 29.8%, $p = 0.004$), had a higher rate of pulmonary complications (33.3% vs 4.7%, $p < 0.001$) and higher chances of kidney failure (13.3% vs 1.4%, $p = 0.002$). Hospital mortality was also greater in this group of patients (20% vs 4.7%, $p = 0.045$). Risk factors associated with this mortality were age ($p = 0.008$), perforated acute diverticulitis with generalized peritonitis ($p = 0.007$), emergency surgery ($p = 0.001$) and a C reactive protein of >20mg/dl ($p = 0.049$). They concluded that both mortality and morbidity of acute diverticulitis is significantly higher in immunocompromised patients. They recommended early diagnosis and early treatment and also recommended considering elective prophylactic sigmoidectomy in those patients with a history of past episodes of acute diverticulitis and in those who are on a waiting list for a transplant surgery. This prophylactic surgery would be crucial to prevent the death of patient, taking into account, of course, their individual risk factors and the best time to perform the surgery.

Klarenbeek et al. [10] described certain risk factors associated with perforation during an episode of acute diverticulitis which included patients with ASA scale of greater than II ($p = 0.041$), patients on immunosuppressive therapy ($p = 0.006$), those with chronic kidney failure ($p = 0.000$) and collagen vascular disease ($p = 0.007$). Having one or more of these risk factors proved to increase the risk of perforation by fivefold (36% vs 7%, $p = 0.002$). Keeping all of this in mind, they recommend considering elective prophylactic sigmoidectomy in these complex cases as they have a high risk of perforation. Similar recommendations have been made by Al Harakeha et al. [22].

Al-Khamis et al. [21] described in their study that a higher proportion of immunocompromised patients who underwent emergency surgery needed a Hartman's procedure, compared to immunocompetent patients (91.4% vs 78.6%, $p < 0.001$). They also reported that laparoscopic procedures were more common among immunocompetent patients (8.5% vs 3.9%, $p < 0.001$). Immunocompromised patients had a higher morbidity rate (45% vs 28%, $p < 0.001$), and the mortality was four times higher after emergency colectomy (16% vs 4%, $p < 0.001$). These patients also had higher rates of wound dehiscence (5.4% vs 3%, $p = 0.002$) and infectious complications

(36% vs 26%, $p < 0.001$). However, no significant differences were found in rate of surgical site infection. Regarding elective colectomy after an episode of acute diverticulitis, immunocompromised patients had a higher proportion of stomas (29.2% vs 10.5%, $p < 0.001$), while as laparoscopic surgery was performed more frequently in immunocompetent patients (58.2% vs 38.2%, $p < 0.001$). Postoperative morbidity and mortality rates were relatively low in both groups, although they were significantly higher in immunocompromised patients, which included surgical site infection, organ infection, dehiscence, pneumonia, re-intubation, kidney failure, cardiac arrest, need for blood transfusion, deep vein thrombosis, sepsis, septic shock, emergency surgery, days of admission and death. In conclusion, immunocompromised patients have significantly higher mortality rates after emergency surgery, but not as much after elective surgery. Therefore, they consider that elective prophylactic surgery should be offered to immunocompromised patients after an episode of acute diverticulitis to avoid a possible emergency surgery, but also considering that morbidity is higher in this group. They recommend new studies to be carried out to identify risk factors for recurrence, making it possible to better select the patients who would benefit from elective surgery.

Scotti et al. [43] analyzed patients with a kidney *transplant* who suffer with a complicated acute diverticulitis, and concluded that emergency surgery had a high mortality rate. Elective surgery, however, had mortality and morbidity rates similar to those of the general population. They recommend a high degree of suspicion for an early diagnosis and early treatment, performing emergency surgery if there is no improvement during the first 48 hours. Hartmann's procedure is their recommended option. They also recommend that elective prophylactic sigmoidectomy should be considered before the transplant in patients with known diverticulosis, those with autosomal dominant polycystic disease or in those with a history of past acute diverticulitis with good evolution after conservative management.

The review by Hwang et al. [9] concluded that the incidence of acute diverticulitis in patients with transplant and those on chronic corticoid treatment is relatively high. They also reported that the mortality rate is greater than that of the general population in these patients. With the current published information, they cannot assume that whether the risk of screening for diverticulosis and performing prophylactic sigmoidectomy is lower than the risk of developing an episode of acute diverticulitis in these patients [9].

CONCLUSION

As previously explained, treatment of acute diverticulitis in immunocompetent patients has changed during past several years. Surgical management during an episode of acute diverticulitis was mandatory and uncontested during the first half of the 20th century. However, today surgery is a last resort during the management of acute diverticulitis, as long as there is no free perforation, sepsis and/or peritonitis. There is still great controversy on the management of acute diverticulitis in immunocompromised patients, as the analyzed studies discussed above have shown. Each study had its own conclusions, based on their results.

If we analyze the conclusions of the 9 more representative studies discussed in this chapter, their recommendations can even be found to be opposing. None of them seem to reach to any conclusions with enough evidence to make any universal recommendations, and all of them recommend new studies to help understand which will be the best management for these complex patients.

Samdani et al. [41] were not able to recommend emergency surgery during the episode of acute diverticulitis, nor a prophylactic elective surgery to prevent more severe recurrences. Biondo et al. [12, 20] only recommend close follow-up during the first year after the first episode of acute diverticulitis in immunocompromised patients. This follow-up should be performed with a high degree of suspicion for recurrences.

Brandl et al. [40] do recommend considering an elective prophylactic sigmoidectomy in patients waiting for a transplant surgery and those with previous history of acute diverticulitis. This consideration should be made taking into account the patient's individual risk factors.

The studies of Klarenbeek et al. [10] and Al Harakeha et al. [22] also recommend elective prophylactic sigmoidectomy in those complex cases which have a higher chance of perforation. Patients with this higher risk are those on immunosuppression drugs, patients with chronic kidney disease or collagen vascular disease. Of course, they recommend more studies to be able to better extrapolate these recommendations.

Al-Khamis et al. [21] described a higher mortality in emergency surgery for immunocompromised patients, but a similar mortality in the general population in elective surgery. They also described a higher morbidity in elective surgery for immunocompromised patients. They recommend further studies to identify risk factors for developing severe acute diverticulitis. Knowing these risk factors would help to make a better selection of immunocompromised patients to be planned for elective surgery, thereby making the morbidity of the surgery acceptable when compared to the mortality of emergency surgery. Scotti et al. [43] recommend elective prophylactic sigmoidectomy in patients on a waiting list for transplant surgery, in those with autosomal dominant polycystic disease and in those with a good evolution after conservative management of a first episode of acute diverticulitis.

If we compare those studies that recommend elective prophylactic surgery and those that do not recommend it, we are not able to make any conclusions or recommendations. Four studies recommend considering elective prophylactic surgery in selected patients, and another four don't recommend it. The ninth study only recommends further studies to better assess the risk factors useful for a more apt selection of patients that could benefit from an elective prophylactic surgery with an acceptable morbidity.

No recommendations for immunocompromised patients with acute diverticulitis can be given after this review. Management of the episode of acute diverticulitis is similar to that of immunocompetent patients. Elective prophylactic surgery can be recommended in selected cases with a higher risk of developing severe acute diverticulitis, such as patients on immunosuppression treatment, those with chronic kidney disease, collagen vascular disease, patients on a wait list for transplant or patients with autosomal dominant polycystic disease.

REFERENCES

[1] Parra, A. and Nicolas, D. (2012). Diverticular disease of the colon. *https://www.aegastro.es/sites/default/files/archivos/ayudaspracticas/38_Enfermedad_diverticular.pdf.*

[2] Von Rahden, B. H. and Germer, C. T. (2012). Pathogenesis of Colonic Diverticular Disease. Langenbeck's *Archives of Surgery*, 397 (7): 1025-1033. doi:10.1007/s00423-012-0961-5.

[3] Liu, P. H., Cao, Y., Keeley, B. R., Tam, I., Wu, K., Strate, L. L., et al. (2017). Adherence to a Healthy Lifestyle is Associated With a Lower Risk of Diverticulitis among Men. *Am J Gastroenterol.*, 112(12): 1868–76.

[4] Strate, L. L., Liu, Y. L., Syngal, S., Aldoori, W. H. and Giovannucci, E. L. (2008). Nut, corn, and popcorn consumption and the incidence of diverticular disease. *JAMA*, 300(8): 907–14.

[5] Aldoori, W. H., Giovannucci, E. L., Rimm, E. B., Wing A. L., Trichopoulos, D. V. and Willett, W. C. (1995). A prospective study of alcohol, smoking, caffeine, and the risk of symptomatic diverticular disease in men. *Ann Epidemiol.*, 5(3):221–8.

[6] Strate, L. L, Liu, Y. L., Huang, E. S., Giovannucci, E. L. and Chan, A. T. (2011). Use of aspirin or nonsteroidal antiinflammatory drugs increases risk for diverticulitis and diverticular bleeding. *Gastroenterology*, 140(5):1427–33.

[7] Maguire, L. H., Song, M., Strate, L. E., Giovannucci, E. L. and Chan, A. T. (2013). Higher serum levels of vitamin D are associated with a reduced risk of diverticulitis. *Clin Gastroenterol Hepatol.*, 11(12): 1631–5.

[8] Feingold, D., Steele, S. R, and Lee, S., (2014). Practice parameters for the treatment of sigmoid diverticulitis. *Dis Colon Rectum,* 57:284–94.

[9] Hwang, S. S., Cannom, R. R., Abbas, M. A., et al. (2010).Diverticulitis in transplant patients and patients on chronic corticosteroid therapy: a systematic review. *Dis Colon Rectum*, 53:1699–707.

[10] Klarenbeek, B. R., Samuels, M., van der Wal, M. A., et al. (2010). Indications for elective sigmoid resection in diverticular disease. *Ann Surg.*, 251 (4):670–4. doi: 10.1097/SLA.0b013e3181d3447d.

[11] Shahedi, K., Fuller, G., Bolus, R., Cohen, E., Vu, M., Shah, R., et al. (2013). Long-term risk of acute diverticulitis among patients with incidental diverticulosis found during colonoscopy. *Clin Gastroenterol Hepatol.*, 11(12):1609–13.

[12] Biondo, S., Borao, J. L. and Kreisler, E. (2012). Recurrence and virulence of colonic diverticulitis in immunocompromised patients. *Am J Surg.*, 204:172–9.

[13] Golda, T., Kreisler, E. and Mercader, C. (2014). Emergency surgery for perforated diverticulitis in the immunosuppressed patient. *Colorectal Dis.*, 16:723–31.

[14] Etzioni, D. A., Mack, T. M. and Beart Jr, R. W. (2009). Diverticulitis in the United States: 1998-2005: changing patterns of disease and treatment. *Ann Surg.*, 249:210–7.

[15] Salem, L., Anaya, D. A. and Roberts, K. E. (2005). Hartmann'scolectomy and reversal in diverticulitis: a population-level assessment. *Dis Colon Rectum*, 48:988–95.

[16] Ludeman, L., Warren, B. F. and Shepherd, N. A.. (2002). The pathology of diverticular disease. *Best Pract Res Clin Gastroenterol,*, 16:543-62.

[17] Elta, G. H. (2004). Urgent colonoscopy for acute lower-GI bleeding. *Gastrointest Endosc.*, 59:402-8.

[18] Kaiser, A. M., Jiang, J. K. and Lake, J. P. (2005). The management of complicated diverticulitis and the role of computed tomography. *Am J Gastroenterol,*, 100(4):910-7.

[19] Hinchey, E. J., Schaal, P. G. and Richards, G. K. (1978). Treatment of perforated diverticular disease of the colon. *Adv Surg.*, 12:85-109.

[20] Biondo, S., Trenti, L., Elvira, J., Golda, T. and Kreisler, E. (2016). Outcomes of colonic diverticulitis according to the reason of immunosuppression. *Am J Surg.*, 212(3): 384–390. Published online May 7. doi: 10.1016/j.amjsurg.2016.01.038.

[21] Al-Khamis, A., Abou Khalil, J., Demian, M., Morin, N., Vasilevsky, C. A., Gordon, P. H. and Boutros, M. (2016). Sigmoid Colectomy for Acute Diverticulitis in Immuno-suppressed vs Immuno-competent Patients: Outcomes from the ACS-NSQIP Database. *Dis Colon Rectum,* 59(2): 101–109. doi: 10.1097/DCR.0000000000000513.

[22] Al Harakeha, H., Pailyb, A. J., Doughana, S. and Shaikhb, I. (2018). Recurrent Acute Diverticulitis: When to Operate?. *Inflamm Intest Dis.*, 3:91–99. www.karger.com/iid doi: 10.1159/000494973.

[23] Rose, J., Parina, R. P., Faiz, O., Chang, D. C. and Talamini, M. A. (2015). Long-term Outcomes After Initial Presentation of Diverticulitis. *Ann Surg.,* 262(6):1046–53.

[24] Humes, D. J., Solaymani-Dodaran, M. and Fleming, K. M.(2009). A population- based study of perforated diverticular disease incidence and associated mortality. *Gastroenterology.*, 136:1198–205.

[25] Larson, E. S., Khalil, H. A. and Lin, A. Y. (2014). Diverticulitis occurs early after lung transplantation. *J Surg Res.*, 190: 667–71.

[26] Qasabian, R. A., Meagher, A. P. and Lee, R.. (2004). Severe diverticulitis after heart, lung, and heart-lung transplantation. *J Heart Lung Transplant.*, 23:845–9.

[27] Sawyerr, O. I., Garvin, P. J., Codd, J. E., Graff, R. J., Newton, W. T. and Willman, V. L. (1978). Colorectal complications of renal allograft transplantation. *Arch Surg.*, 113:84 – 86.

[28] McCune, T. R., Nylander, W.A. and Van Buren, DH.(1992). Colonic screening prior to renal transplantation and its impact on post-transplant colonic complications. *Clin Transplant,*, 6:91– 96.

[29] Pourfarziani, V., Mousavi-Nayeeni, S. M.and Ghaheri, H.(2007). The outcome of diverticulosis in kidney recipients with polycystic kidney disease. *Transplant Proc.*, 39:1054 –1056.

[30] Perkins, J. D., Shield, C.F. 3rd, Chang, F. C., and Farha, G. J. (1984). Acute diverticulitis: comparison of treatment in immunocompromised and non-immunocompromised patients. *Am J Surg.*, 148:745– 748.

[31] Soravia, C., Baldi, A. and Kartheuser, A. (1995). Acute colonic complications after kidney transplantation. *Acta Chir Belg.*, 95:157–161.

[32] Lederman, E. D., Conti, D. J,. Lempert, N., Singh, T. P. and Lee, E. C. (1998). Complicated diverticulitis following renal transplantation. *Dis Colon Rectum,* 41:613– 618.

[33] Khan, S., Eppstein, A. C. and Anderson, G. K. (2001). Acute diverticulitis in heart and lung transplant patients. *Transpl Int.*, 14:12–15.

[34] Dalla Valle, R., Capocasale, E. and Mazzoni, M. P. (2005). Acute diverticulitis with colon perforation in renal transplantation. *Transplant Proc.*, 37:2507–2510.

[35] Hutchinson, D., and Lynch, M. (2001). Sigmoide diverticular abscess perforation in 2 patients with rheumatoid arthritis treated with high dose corticosteroids: a cautionary tale. *J Rheumatol,*, 28: 1935–1936.

[36] Domínguez Fernández, E., Albrecht, K. H. and Heemann, U. (1998). Prevalence of diverticulosis and incidence of bowel perforation after kidney transplantation in patients with polycystic kidney disease. *Transpl Int.*, 11:28 –31.

[37] Beaver, T. M., Fullerton, D. A. and Zamora, M. R.. (1996). Colon perforation after lung transplantation. *Ann Thorac Surg.*, 62: 839 – 843.

[38] Fenton, J. J. and Cicale, M. J. (1997). Sigmoid diverticular perforation complicating lung transplantation. *J Heart Lung Transplant.*, 16: 681–685.

[39] Carson, S. D., Krom, R. A., Uchida, K., Yokota, K., West, J. C. and Weil, R. 3rd. (1978). Colon perforation after kidney transplantation. *Ann Surg.*, 188:109 –113.

[40] Brandl, A., Kratzer, T., Kafka-Ritsch, R., Braunwarth, E., Denecke, C., Weiss, S., Atanasov, G., Sucher, R., Biebl, M., Aigner, F., Pratschke, J., Öllinger, R. and Can, J. (2016). Diverticulitis in immunosuppressed patients: A fatal outcome requiring a new approach? *Surg.*, 59(4): 254–261. doi: 10.1503/cjs.012915.

[41] Samdani, T., Pieracci, F. M., Eachempati, S. R., Benarroch-Gampel, J., Weiss, A., Pietanza, M. C., Barie, P. S. and Nash, G. M. (2014). Colonic diverticulitis in chemotherapy patients: should operative

indications change? A retrospective cohort study. *Int J Surg.*, 12(12):1489-94. doi: 10.1016/j.ijsu.2014.10.032.

[42] Machado, T. C. and Malheiro, L. S. (2017). The role of elective surgery following acute colonic diverticulitis. *Revista Portuguesa de Cirurgia*, (40), 21-33. [Portuguese Journal of Surgery, (40), 21-33.].

[43] Scotti, A., Santangelo, M., Federico, S., Carrano, R., La Tessa, C., Carlomagno, N., Palmieri, D. G., Calogero, A., Piantadosi, M. and Renda, A. (2014). Complicated diverticulitis in kidney transplanted patients: Analysis of 717 cases. *Transplant Proc.*, 46(7): 2247–2250. doi: 10.1016/j.transproceed.2014.07.044.

In: Diverticulitis: Diagnosis and Treatment ISBN: 978-1-53618-081-7
Editors: Shams-ul-Bari et al.

Chapter 6

MANAGEMENT OF COMPLICATED DIVERTICULITIS

Shams ul Bari*
Department of Surgery, Skims Medical College, Srinagar, Kashmir, India

ABSTRACT

The term diverticulitis refers to inflammation of one or more diverticula. It includes a spectrum of diseases ranging from mild localized inflammation to a severe inflammation resulting into a free perforation and generalized peritonitis. In uncomplicated diverticulitis, diverticula and the surrounding intestinal lining are inflamed but there are no signs of pus or any sign of spreading inflammation. In complicated diverticulitis the inflammation has already spread and there is abscess formation and even intestinal perforation. Complications develop in only 20% patients of patients with diverticulitis, while as in remaining 80% of patients, diverticulitis resolves without any serious complications.

Patients with diverticulitis should be ideally hospitalized for treatment and for close observation. Initially all the patients should be put on conservative line of management which includes intravenous fluid therapy, nasogastric suction and broad spectrum intravenous antibiotics. Patients

* Corresponding Author's Email: shamsulbari@rediffmail.com, shamsulbari1@gmail.com.

who fail to show response within 48 hours usually need some intervention. Approximately 20% patients who develop acute diverticulitis, may develop complications and will need some surgical intervention. The absolute indications for surgical intervention include peritonitis, abscess formation, fistula formation, obstruction, intractable haemorrhage and inability to exclude carcinoma. The type of surgical treatment depends on the severity and extent of underlying disease and may include resection of involved segment and primary anastomosis or resection of the involved segment with colostomy.

INTRODUCTION

Complicated diverticulitis is defined as diverticulitis associated with abscess formation phlegmon, fistula, obstruction, bleeding, or perforation [1-11]. Complicated diverticulitis is a significant cause of morbidity and mortality in patients suffering from diverticulitis. An overall mortality rates of 6% and 17% has been reported after surgery for complicated diverticulitis [1-11]. Perforated diverticulitis is associated with significantly higher mortality and morbidity rates. The mortality rates of 22% and 39% have been reported following free perforation and fecal peritonitis in complicated diverticulitis [10-12]. Some studies have reported that perforation may be the first manifestation of complicated diverticulitis in as many as 50% to 70% patients [1, 2, 4, 5].

Prophylactic surgery has been recommended by large number of authors to prevent serious complications of recurrent colonic diverticulitis. [2, 7, 12-16]. This recommendation is based on the fact that complicated diverticulitis usually develops after multiple episodes of diverticulitis [2, 4, 15-18] Elective resections have been associated with a low mortality rate of between 1% and 4% [2, 5, 16]. After one episode of diverticulitis recurrence rate of more than 40% has been reported in literature with complications occurring in 30% to 40% of patients [7, 17-19]. After a second attack of diverticulitis, the incidence of complications may be as high as 50% to 60%, while as the mortality rate may be twice the mortality rate associated with initial attack. Thus, the practice of prophylactic surgery is being followed on the observation that (a) episodes of diverticulitis often recur and may run a complicated course, (b) all patients are at risk for a perforated diverticulitis after first episode, and (c) the risk of recurrent diverticulitis and colostomy is eliminated with elective surgical intervention. Therefore it is better to practice elective colon resection after 2 episodes of non-complicated diverticulitis rather than to wait for inevitable perforation with septic complications, once the patient has had 2 or more attacks of diverticulitis [18-25].

Diagnosis of Complicated Diverticulitis

Ultrasonography is a simple and very useful diagnostic tool for diagnosis of complicated diverticulitis, although its usefulness depends on the experience of the sonologist [13, 14, 15, 16]. However, Computed tomography is considered as the investigation of choice for diagnosis of suspected cases of complicated diverticulitis and has got a sensitivity of 95-97% and a specificity of 100% [9, 10, 11]. Computed tomography is minimally invasive, rapid, and widely available. It not only helps in diagnosis, but is a vital tool for follow up of the patients [12]. It gives an accurate information about the size, number and location of an abscesses. It also provides an objective analysis of the severity of the diverticulitis. It is on the basis of CT finding that the treatment options are decided [26, 27].

Classification of Complicated Diverticulitis

Complicated diverticulitis has been traditionally classified into four stages on the basis of Hinchey classification [17] and is being widely used till date for determining the treatment strategy for complicated diverticulitis. However in the recent past this classification has been considered increasingly unsuitable as other advanced imaging modalities have become available and because of improvements in conservative management. Currently a modified versions of the Hinchey classification is being used widely in clinical practice [28].

Hinchey Classification

The four clinical stages of perforated diverticular disease are as under [17, 18, 28]:

- Stage I is a pericolic abscess confined by the mesentery of the colon.
- Stage II is a pelvic abscess resulting from local perforation of a pericolic abscess.
- Stage III is a generalized peritonitis resulting from the rupture of either a pericolic or a pelvic abscess into the general peritoneal cavity.
- Stage IV is a fecal peritonitis resulting from the free perforation of a diverticulum.

A modified Hinchey classification was proposed by Kaiser et al., in 2005 [18, 28], wherein the size and range of abscess formation, perforated diverticulitis and the severity of peritonitis are taken into account. These authors introduced stage 0, and divided stage I into stage Ia and stage 1b. In stage 1a, there is a limited pericolic inflammation and while as in stage Ib, there is an abscess formation. In 2011, Dharmarajan et al., [19] reported a new CT grading system for perforated diverticulitis that considers the amount and location of extra luminal air and the size of the abscess. Any abscess of >4 cm requires percutaneous drainage, whereas smaller abscesses can be treated with antibiotic therapy alone (Siewert et al., 20).

Modified Hinchey Classification

Based on the modified Hinchey classification, diverticulitis may be categorized into six stages (0, Ia, Ib, II, III, IV).

- Stage 0; clinically mild diverticulitis
- Stage I; Pericolic abscess or phlegmon formation

- Stage Ia; Confined pericolic inflammation and phlegmonous inflammation
- Stage Ib; Abscess formation (<5 cm) in the proximity of the primary inflammatory process
- Stage II; Pelvic, intra-abdominal, or retroperitoneal abscess
- Stage III; Generalized purulent peritonitis
- Stage IV; Generalized fecal peritonitis.

Computed Tomography Staging of Diverticulitis

According to Kaiser et al., [27], Computed tomography (CT) findings seen in diverticulitis can be divided into following six stages.

- Stage 0; Diverticula with or without wall thickening of the colon
- Stage Ia; Colonic wall thickening with inflammatory reaction in pericolic fatty tissue
- Stage Ib; Stage Ia + pericolic or mesocolic abscess formation
- Stage II; Stage Ia + distant abscess formation (mostly pelvic or interloop abscesses)
- Stage III; Free air with local or generalized free fluid and possible thickening of the peritoneum, there is no open communication with bowel lumen.
- Stage IV; Free perforation, with open communication with bowel lumen.

Indications of Surgery in Complicated Diverticulitis and Their Management

The development of complicated diverticulitis increases with age and has been estimated to develop in approximately one third of patients who have a history of acute diverticulitis [19-22]. Septic complications such as abscess formation, free perforation and peritonitis are the most common complications which need surgical intervention. The other complications of diverticulitis which need surgical intervention include recurrent attacks, fistula formation, obstruction, intractable haemorrhage, chronic stricture, persistent abdominal pain or abdominal mass and inability to exclude carcinoma [29, 30]. Each of these complications may coexist at any given point of time. Surgical intervention is also needed in young patients less than 40 years in age, those with right sided diverticulitis, patients on corticosteroids, those who are immunocompromised and those who don't respond to medical treatment. Although in 80% of people diverticulitis remains uncomplicated, about 20% develop some type of complication [12, 29, 32] and surgical intervention is necessary in almost all these patients. The distribution of different complications for which surgical intervention needed include abscess formation (40-50%), intestinal obstruction (10-15%), free perforation (10-15%) and fistula formation (4-10%).

Abscess Formation

The inflammation is usually localized to the area adjacent to the perforation, thus forming pericolic abscess. About 20% of patients with diverticulitis develop a localized abscess at a pericolonic site (stage Ib) or in the pelvis or retroperitoneal space (stage II). These diverticular abscesses are extremely common and according to location they could be peridiverticular, retroperitoneal, mesenteric or pelvic. Sometimes the abscess can spread to adjacent structures and may present as anterior abdominal wall, hip or thigh abscess. In some cases, liver abscess may develop as a secondary complication of this disease. The patient usually presents with pain, fever, leukocytosis and mass with tenderness may be elicited on per abdominal, pelvic and rectal examination.

With localised peritonitis, medical treatment is justified with careful observation of the patient. When the acute inflammation has subsided completely, patients can be taken for elective operation. However adequate local drainage of pus, primary resection of the segment with end colostomy and mucous fistula is considered as the most appropriate option. Conservative treatment using broad spectrum antibiotics is successful in more than 70% patients with abscess size smaller than 4 cm. Preoperative percutaneous drainage under Usg guidance or CT guidance has also been reported in literature and has been recognized as a standard therapeutic approach. It should be attempted if the conservative management fails or abscess size is more than 4 cm. The argument is that it helps to stabilize the critically ill patients so that they can be taken for elective one stage resection of the diseased colon at later stage. Advocates of this option are of the opinion that sepsis can be controlled in more than 80% of patients. However since the underlying focus of infection is not removed, surgeon should be cautious while choosing this option [30-33]. However, Percutaneous drainage is often difficult when there are small bowel loops adjacent to the fluid collection. In some of these patients, transluminal endoscopic approach through the perforated diverticulum can be attempted, which is an easy, safe and effective method for draining such an abscess cavity [23]. By this method, the risk of damage to the intestinal loop surrounding the abscess is reduced and the drainage route is generally shorter than that of the trans-abdominal route. However, in all these cases of diverticulitis, surgical option should always be kept in mind [8]. An elective surgery can be planned 6 weeks later after drainage of abscess wherein removal of the entire diseased, brittle colon should be done.

Free Perforation and Peritonitis

Perforated diverticulitis is very often the first manifestation of complicated diverticular disease and carries the highest risk of mortality and morbidity. It is not known exactly who are the patients who are at risk for the development of perforated diverticulitis as the initial manifestation of diverticular disease. Although many studies have concluded that those patients whor are immunocompromised are at higher risk for developing perforated diverticulitis. Most of the episodes of perforated diverticulitis are confined to peri-diverticular area or pelvis, but some patients may present with features of generalized peritonitis. Approximately 6% of patients develop severe diverticulitis with perforation and generalized peritonitis (Stage III - stage IV). This diffuse contamination of the peritoneal cavity may occur secondary to rupture of inflamed diverticulum or rupture of pericolic abscess into the free peritoneal cavity. Rarely in some patients, the initial perforation is not walled off, as a result of which free perforation occurs resulting into generalized peritonitis. The overall mortality may be as high as 20-40% due to septic shock and multiple organ failure. Patient with generalized peritonitis need urgent emergency treatment. Several options are available for managing these patients. Since bowel preparation is not possible in emergency situation, two stage or three stage procedure is advocated. One option is thorough irrigation of the peritoneal cavity, closure of the perforation and proximal diverting colostomy. In less infective cases, where colon can be safely mobilized, resection of the diseased segment, end to end primary anastomosis, and proximal decompressing colostomy is performed. In the third option diseased bowel is resected, the proximal bowel is brought out as end colostomy. The distal end may be either brought out as mucous fistula or it may be closed and left in situ as a Hartmann procedure. In all these procedures peritoneal cavity is thoroughly irrigated and drains are left. The colostomy is closed after 8 to 12 weeks. The three stage procedure consists of drainage and thorough lavage of peritoneal cavity, drainage of the involved segment along with creation of a proximal diverting colostomy. After about 3-6 months, resection of diseased segment is carried along with end to end anastomosis. In the third step, proximal colostomy is than closed after 6-8 weeks. Several studies have reported that primary resection can be carried out safely with a morbidity of 25% to 30% and mortality of 5% to 10%. On the other hand morbidity of 50% and mortality of 30% has been reported with simple drainage of abscess with proximal diverting colostomy [7, 19, 29, 32]. Simple drainage with proximal colostomy should be carried out only in those patients where diseased colon is densely adherent to adjacent structures such as ureter, urinary bladder or iliac vessels. In all other cases, resection of the diseased segment should be attempted.

Obstruction

Obstruction is a less common complication of chronic diverticulitis. Such obstruction is usually Partial or incomplete. The obstruction may be due to stricture formation secondary to chronic inflammation. It may also be because of spasm or edema with an element of associated paralytic ileus. Sometimes obstruction may be complete due to repeated episodes with a resultant fibrosis and stenosis. Occasionally a loop of small bowel may become densely adherent due to inflammation of the colon, with a subsequent small bowel obstruction. X-ray abdomen in a standing position is a very useful investigation to differentiate between small and large bowel obstruction. Resection of the diseased bowel with either primary anastomosis or colostomy should be done depending on the severity of disease and adequacy of bowel preparation.

Fistulization

Fistula formation is a rare complication of diverticulitis and may be seen in 4% to 20% patients with diverticular disease. The fistula formation could be internal and very rarely external. Internal fistulas may be seen in as many as 5% cases between the involved segment and the adjacent structures such as urinary bladder, ileum, uterus, vagina and ureter. The most common site for fistulization is the sigmoid colon as it is involved in more than 90% cases of diverticulitis. As far as the incidence of internal fistula formation is concerned, Colovesical fistula is the most common type of fistula and accounts for up to two-thirds of all the internal diverticular fistulas, followed by colocutaneous fistulas, colovaginal and coloenteric fistulas in decreasing order. Although spontaneous external fistulas (colocutaneous fistulas) are rare, but occur postoperatively through incision or drainage site. Other fistulas such as between colon and ureter and colon and uterus are very rare.

Diverticulitis is the most common cause of colovesical fistulas followed by malignancy, inflammatory bowel disease, and radiation therapy. Fistula formation occurs because of direct extension of a ruptured diverticulum or erosion of a peridiverticular abscess into the bladder. Colovesical fistula has been reported to be three to five times more common in males as compared to females. This is because of presence of uterus, which acts as an anatomic barrier between colon and bladder in females. This is why that history of hysterectomy is seen in more than 60% of female who develop Colovesical fistula secondary to diverticulitis.

Pneumaturia (air in urine) and faecaluria (faeces in urine) are the two diagnostic clinical features of Colovesical and coloureteric fistulas. Faecaluria is seen in 48% to 75% while as Pneumaturia is seen in 41% to 75% patients [29, 30, 31]. Recurrent urinary tract infection with fever is another common presentation of these patients as dysuria may be seen in as many as 29% to 75% of patients with Colovesical fistula [32, 33].

Although Pneumaturia and faecaluria are the two diagnostic clinical features of Colovesical and colo-ureteric fistulas, further investigation are needed to confirm the diagnosis. Cystoscopy and barium enema are the ideal investigation for confirming the presence of a Colovesical fistula and its likely cause. Cystoscopy and cystography has got the diagnostic accuracy of 80% to 90% and can demonstrate fistula in 20% of the patients. However, localized inflammation and bullous edema of the bladder mucosa are the most common findings reported on cystoscopy. Findings on barium enema are nonspecific although actual fistula can be seen in as many as 30% patients. Other investigations which are useful in these patients include sigmoidoscopy, colonoscopy and computed tomography. Out of these, CT scan abdomen with an oral contrast has got the better diagnostic value as it can also give information about the extent of disease outside the colon and the urinary bladder [18, 29, 30]. CT is the preferable diagnostic imaging modality due to its high sensitivity of more than 90%). Fistulas may be demonstrated by the presence of gas or contrast in the bladder, or local colonic and bladder wall thickening. CT also helps to assess the degree of pelvic inflammation and to determine optimal timing for surgery. Magnetic resonance imaging (MRI) is another diagnostic modality nowadays available for evaluation of patients with Colovesical fistula. Although highly sensitive, it is expensive and less accessible [30].

Operative procedure is to be performed in all patients with the diagnosis of colovesical fistula [33-39]. Since the disease has been there for a quite a long time, patients can be prepared for elective one stage operative procedures. One stage operation can be performed safely in 90% patients with a colovesical fistula of diverticular origin. Patients are subjected to proper preoperative preparation which includes use of both oral and sytemic antibiotics as well as mechanical preparation. In case of colovesical disease, fistula in urinary bladder is dissected out and the bladder wall is closed, diseased colon is resected and primary anastomosis is performed. The mortality of up to 5% has been reported with colovesical fistula [41-45]. In patients with colouterine fistula, hysterectomy with resection of involved colon and primary anastomosis is carried out. In case of coloenetric fistula, segment of ileum and the diseased bowel is resected followed by primary anastomosis. When inflammatory process is too extensive, operation is performed in two stages. In the first stage, the diseased bowel is resected and the proximal colon is brought as an end colostomy, while the distal end is closed. Anastomosis is carried out at later stage. In more severe cases of inflammation, proximal diverting colostomy is performed in first stage. When the inflammation has subsided, an adequate resection is performed and end to end anastomosis is done.

Management of the Bladder in Colo-Vesical Fistula Repair

There are no acceptable guidelines as far as management of the bladder in colovesical fistula repair **is** concerned . Different techniques have been described in literature which include use of an omental patch to close the bladder defect or wedge resection of the affected bladder area with closure using sutures or an omental patch and pinch off technique followed by simple closure [46]. If the defect is small, simple decompression with an indwelling catheter alone may be sufficient [47, 48, 49]. Initial recommendation was that the indwelling catheter should remain in situ for

14 days. However, studies conducted in recent times have not demonstrated any difference between early and late removal of catheter, although prolonged catheterisation is associated with an increased risk of infection. Lynn et al., in his study has found that the risk of recurrence was significantly higher in advanced bladder repairs and the use of ureteric stents has no advantage [50].

Morbidity after Complicated Diverticulitis

Different types of morbidities after complicated diverticulitis that have been reported in literature include anastomotic leak, wound dehiscence, wound infection requiring debridement and intra-abdominal abscess. Cardiac complications, pulmonary complications and partial small bowel obstruction with ileus are the other common causes of postoperative morbidity reported in different studies [51]. Older age, cirrhosis, steroid use, chemotherapy, preexisting comorbidities, and perforated diverticulitis are all significantly associated with increased postoperative morbidity [52].

Many studies have shown a significant correlation between immunosuppression and perforation as well as poor outcomes [11, 31, 32]. Postoperative morbidity and mortality has been reported as high as 65% and 39% in the immunocompromised patients as compared to 24% and 2% in immune-competent patients. There is a consensus that immuno-compromised patients, including elderly patients, should be taken for early sigmoid resection to avoid perforation peritonitis and subsequent increased morbidity and mortality.

References

[1] Berry A. R., and Turner W. H.(1989). Emergency surgery for complicated diverticular disease: a five year experience. *Dis Colon Rectum,* 32:849-854. [PubMed] [Google Scholar].

[2] Hackford A. W. and Schoetz D. J.(1985). Surgical management of complicated diverticulitis: the Lahey Clinic experience, 1967 to 1982. *Dis Colon Rectum*, 28:317-321. [PubMed] [Google Scholar].

[3] Wedell J. and Banzhaf G.(1997). Surgical management of complicated colonic diverticulitis. *Br J Surg,* 84: 380-383. [PubMed] [Google Scholar].

[4] Lambert M. E. and Knox R. A.(1986). Management of the septic complications of diverticular disease. *Br J Surg,* 73: 576-579. [PubMed] [Google Scholar].

[5] Rodkey G. E. and Welch C. E.(1984). Changing patterns in the surgical treatment of diverticular disease. *Ann Surg,* 200: 466-477. [PMC free article] [PubMed] [Google Scholar].

[6] Nylamo E.(1990). Diverticulitis of the colon: role of surgery in preventing complications. *Ann Chirurgiae et Gynaecologiae,* 79: 139-142. [PubMed] [Google Scholar].

[7] Chappius C. W. and Cohn I. Jr.(1988).Acute colonic diverticulitis. *Surg Clin North Am,* 68:301-312. [PubMed] [Google Scholar].

[8] Farmakis N., Tudor R. G. and Keighley M. R.(1994). The 5-year natural history of complicated diverticular disease. *Br J Surg,* 81: 733-735. [PubMed] [Google Scholar].

[9] Schwesinger W. H. and Page C. P.(2000). Operative management of diverticular emergencies: strategies and outcomes. *Arch Surg,*135: 558-562. [PubMed] [Google Scholar].

[10] Rothenberger D. A. and Wiltz O.(1993). Surgery for complicated diverticulitis. *Surg Clin North Am,* 73: 975-992. [PubMed] [Google Scholar].

[11] Nagorney D. M., Adson M. A. and Pemberton J. H.(1985). Sigmoid diverticulitis with perforation and generalized peritonitis. *Dis Colon Rectum,* 28:71-75. [PubMed] [Google Scholar].

[12] Marshall S. F.(1963).Earlier resection in one stage for diverticulitis of the colon. *Am Surg,*29: 337-346. [Google Scholar].

[13] Tyau E. S. and Prystowsky J. B.(1991). Acute diverticulitis: a complicated problem in the immunocompromised patient. *Arch Surg,* 126:855-859. [PubMed] [Google Scholar].

[14] Kronborg O.(1993). Treatment of perforated sigmoid diverticulitis: a prospective randomized trial. *Br J Surg,* 80:505-507. [PubMed] [Google Scholar].

[15] Griffen W. O.Jr.(1976). Management of the acute complications of diverticular disease: acute perforation of colonic diverticula. *Dis Colon Rectum.* 1976; 19:293-295. [PubMed] [Google Scholar].

[16] Wong W. D. and Wexner S. D.(2000) Practice parameters for the treatment of sigmoid diverticulitis - supporting documentation. *Dis Colon Rectum,* 43: 289-297. [PubMed] [Google Scholar].

[17] Boles R. S. Jr. and Jordan S. M.(1958) The clinical significance of diverticulosis. *Gastroenterology,* 35:579. [PubMed] [Google Scholar].

[18] Colcock B. P.(1958) Surgical management of complicated diverticulitis. *N Engl J Med,* 259: 570. [PubMed] [Google Scholar].

[19] Roberts P., Abel M. and Rosen L.(1995). Practice parameters for sigmoid diverticulitis - supporting documentation. *Dis Colon Rectum,* 38: 126-132. [Google Scholar].

[20] Parks T. G.(1969). Natural history of diverticular disease of the colon. A review of 521 cases. *BMJ,* 639-642. [PMC free article] [PubMed] [Google Scholar].

[21] Schoetz D. J.(1999). Diverticular disease of the colon: a century old problem. *Dis Colon Rectum,* 42: 703-709. [PubMed] [Google Scholar].

[22] Hart A. R., Kennedy J. H. and Stebbings W. S.(2000). How frequently do large bowel diverticula perforate? An incidence and cross-sectional study. *Eur J Gastroenterol Hepatol,* 12: 661-666. [PubMed] [Google Scholar].

[23] Chautems R. C. and Ambrosetti P.(2002). Long-term follow-up after first acute episode of sigmoid diverticulitis: is surgery mandatory? *Dis Colon Rectum,* 45: 962-966. [PubMed] [Google Scholar].

[24] Haglund U. and Hellberg R.(1979). Complicated diverticular disease of the sigmoid colon: an analysis of short and long term outcome in 392 patients. *Ann Chirug et Gynaecologiae,* 68:41-46. [PubMed] [Google Scholar].

[25] Anaya D. A. and Flum D. R.(2004). Assessing the Risk of Emergency Colectomy and Colostomy in Patients with Diverticular Disease. Presented at the *American College of Surgeons 90th Annual Clinical Congress*; New Orleans, LA,October 2004.

[26] Morris J., Stellato, T. A., Hagga, J. R. and Liberman, J.(1986).The utility of computed tomography in Colonc diverticulitis. *Ann. surg,* 204:128.

[27] Kaiser A. M., Jiang J. K. and Lake J. P.(2005). The management of complicated diverticulitis and the role of computed tomography. *Am J Gastroenterol,* 100; 910-917.

[28] Hinchey E. J., Schaal P. G. and Richards G. K.(1978). Treatment of perforated diverticular disease of the colon. *Adv surg,* 12:85-109.

[29] Anthony L. Imbembo.(1997). Diverticular disease of the colon. In: Sebeston D. C., Lyerly H. K., *text book of surgery, the biological basis of modern surgical practice,* 15th edition W. B. Saunders company, 982-993.

[30] Stabile, B. E., Puccio, E., Van sonnenberg, E. and Neff, C.(1990) preoperative percutaneous drainage of diverticular abscess. *Am. j. Surg,* 159:99.

[31] Eng K., Ranson J. H. C. and Locolia S. A.(1977). Resection of the perforated segment; A significant advance in tretamnet of dicerticulitis with free perforation of abscess. *Am. J. Surg,* 133-67.

[32] Labs J. D., Sarr M. G., Fishman E. K., Siegelman S. S. and Cameron J. L.(1988). Complications of acute diverticulitis of colon: Improved early diagnosis with computerised tomography. *Am. j surg,* 155:331.

[33] Letwin E. R.(1982). Diverticulitis of the colon: Clinical review of acute presentation and management. *Am. J. surg*, 143:579.

[34] Netri G. and Verbo A.(2000).The role of surgical treatment in colon diverticulitis: indications and results. *Ann Ital Chir.* 71: 209-214. [PubMed] [Google Scholar].

[35] Killingback M.(2005). Surgical treatment of diverticulitis. In: Fazio V. W., Church J. M., Delaney C. P., eds. *Current Therapy in Colon and Rectal Surgery*, 2nd ed. Elsevier Mosby, 285-295. [Google Scholar].

[36] Benn P. L., Wolff B. G. and Illstrup D. M.(1986). Level of anastomosis and recurrent colonic diverticulitis *Am J Surg*, 151: 269-271. [PubMed] [Google Scholar].

[37] Thorn M., Graf W.(2002).Clinical and functional results after elective colonic resection in 75 consecutive patients with diverticular disease. *Am J Surg*, 183:7-11. [PubMed] [Google Scholar].

[38] Salem L. and Veenstra D. L.(2004).The timing of elective colectomy in diverticulitis: a decision analysis. *J Am Coll Surg,* 199:904-912. [PubMed] [Google Scholar].

[39] Sterioff S., Orringer M. B. and Cameron J. L.(1974).Colon perforations associated with steroid therapy. *Surgery,* 75:56-58. [PubMed] [Google Scholar].

[40] Lederman E. D. and Conti D. J.(1998). Complicated diverticulitis following renal transplantation. *Dis Colon Rectum,* 41:613-618. [PubMed] [Google Scholar].

[41] Haglund U., Hellberg R., Johnsen C. and Hulte L.(1979). Complicated diverticular disease of the sigmoid colon. An analysis of short and long term outcome in 392 patients. *Ann. Chir. Gynaecol,* 68: 41, 1979.

[42] Kirsch G. M., Hampel N., Shuck J. M. and Resnick M. I.(1991). Diagnosis and management of vesicoenteeric fistulas. *Surg. gynecol. obstet,* 173:91.

[43] Woods R. J., Lavery I. C., Fazio V. W., jagelman D. G. and Weakley F. L.(1988). Internal fistulas in diverticular disease. *Dis. colon rectum,* 31:591.

[44] Benn P. L., Wolff B. G. and llstrup D. M.(1986). level of anastomosis and recurrent colonic diverticulitisn. *Am. J. surg,* 151; 269.

[45] Makela J., Kiviniemi H. and Laitinen S.(2002). Prevelance of perforated sigmoid diverticulitis is increasing. *Dis Colon Rectum,* 45: 955-961.

[46] Scozzari G., Arezzo A. and Morino M.(2010). Enterovesical fistulas: diagnosis and management. *Tech Coloproctol,* 14(4):293-300. [PubMed] [Google Scholar].

[47] Mileski W. J., Joehl R. J., Rege R. V. and Nahrwold D. L.(1987). One-stage resection and anastomosis in the management of colovesical fistula. *Am J Surg,* 153(1):75-79. [PubMed] [Google Scholar].

[48] Rao P. N., Knox R., Barnard R. J. and Schofield P. F.(1987). Management of colovesical fistula. *Br J Surg,* 74(4):362-363. [PubMed] [Google Scholar].

[49] Steele M., Deveney C. and Burchell M.(1978). Diagnosis and management of colovesical fistulas. *Dis Colon Rectum,* 22(1):27-30. [PubMed] [Google Scholar].

[50] Schlachta C. M., Mamazza J., Seshadri P. A., Cadeddu M. O. and Poulin EC.(2000). Predicting conversion to open surgery in laparoscopic colorectal resections: a simple clinical model. *Surg Endosc,* 14(12):1114-1117. [PubMed] [Google Scholar].

[51] Chapman J., Davies, M., Wolff B., Dozois E.,Tessier D., Harrington J. and Larson D. (2005). Complicated Diverticulitis; *Ann Surg,* 242(4): 576-583. doi: https://dx.doi.org./10.1097/01.sla.0000184843.89836.35, PMCID: PMC1402355 PMID: 16192818.

[52] Tochigi T., Kosugi C., Shuto K., Mori M., Hirano A.and Koda K. (January, 2018). Management of complicated diverticulitis of the colon. *Annals of Gastroenterological Surgery.* vol. 2 (1): 22-27.

[53] Painter N. S. and Burkitt D. P.(1975). Diverticular disease of the colon.20th century problem. *Clinical gastroeneterol,* 4:3.

In: Diverticulitis: Diagnosis and Treatment ISBN: 978-1-53618-081-7
Editors: Shams-ul-Bari et al.

Chapter 7

LAPAROSCOPIC MANAGEMENT OF DIVERTICULITIS

Shams ul Bari *

Department of surgery, Skims Medical College, Srinagar, Jammu and Kashmir, India

ABSTRACT

Surgical intervention may be required in around 10% patients with diverticulitis. With the increasing experience in laparoscopy, minimally invasive surgery is being widely employed in emergency situations such as generalized peritonitis due to diverticulitis. Multiple prospective studies and retrospective analysis in colorectal surgery have confirmed that the laparoscopic approach provided better outcome than the open approach. The advantages of laparoscopy are less postoperative pain, improved respiratory function, short hospital stay and lowered postoperative morbidities. The laparoscopic approach has been performed in all types of procedures related to complicated diverticular disease, such as Hartman procedure, sigmoid resection with primary anastomosis (RPA) and reversal of HP. Laparoscopic lavage drainage, a previously unknown technique for the management of purulent peritonitis is also gaining acceptance and has

* Corresponding Author's Email: shamsulbari@rediffmail.com.

provided new therapeutic approach in the management of complicated diverticulitis.

Despite worldwide application, a precise consensus has not yet been established to determine the exact status of laparoscopic techniques in complicated diverticulitis. Well-built large randomized controlled trials are necessary to establish the role of Laparoscopy in Hartman procedure, sigmoid resection and anastomosis and generalised peritonitis and to confirm the advantages of laparoscopy in the management of chronic complications of diverticulitis and in reversal of Hartman procedure.

INTRODUCTION

Laparoscopic management of diverticulitis has become widely accepted modality of management for diverticulitis, including anterior resection for recurrent uncomplicated disease and lavage or drainage for purulent peritonitis and abscesses that cannot be drained by percutaneous approach [1, 2, 3]. Multiple prospective studies in colorectal surgery have confirmed the safety and feasibility of laparoscopic approach over the open approach [4-6]. The advantages of laparoscopy being less postoperative pain, improved respiratory function, short hospital stay and lowered postoperative morbidities [19-22]. Based on these advantages, laparoscopy has been considered as the preferred choice for the elective treatment of diverticular disease [1, 11-20]. However, due to insufficient data for confirming validity of laparoscopy, the American Society of Colon and Rectal Surgeons and the European Association of Endoscopic Surgeons have not recommended the routine use of laparoscopy in the emergency situations including the management of complicated perforated diverticulitis [21-25].

However recently due to worldwide increase in experience in colorectal and minimally invasive surgery, the use of laparoscopy in abdominal emergencies has also gained acceptability [26]. Several studies conducted recently have reported the benefits of laparoscopy over the open approach in selected patients with perforated diverticulitis [25, 27-31].

LAPAROSCOPY IN EMERGENCY SURGERY

Almost all procedures for complicated diverticular disease have been performed laparoscopically. The reversal of Hartmann procedure has been progressively performed laparoscopically with less morbidity and mortality [32-34]. Sigmoid colonic resection and primary anastomosis with or without diverting loop ileostomy (DI) has been repeatedly performed in diverticular peritonitis with excellent results [35]. Laparoscopic lavage drainage, a previously unknown technique for the management of purulent peritonitis [36-39] is also gaining acceptance in the management of complicated diverticulitis.

Despite worldwide application, a precise consensus has not yet been established based on the level 1 evidence data, to determine the exact status of laparoscopic techniques in complicated diverticulitis. In a study conducted by Letarte F, et al. [40, 41], outcome of laparoscopic surgery in 24 patients with Hinchey 1 and 2 disease was compared to open surgery in 18 patients. Overall complication rate was four times less, bowel movements were faster, hospital stay was shorter while as operative time was longer in laparoscopy group. Resection with primary anastomosis was possible in all patients except one, while as conversion to open surgery was required in 2 patients. Despite favourable results from this study, randomized controlled studies are needed to confirm the suggested benefits of laparoscopy in this group of patients.

Laparoscopic lavage drainage was first described in 1996 and consists of a laparoscopic exploration of the abdominal cavity followed by lavage with heated saline serum and drainage of the diseased colon for the next several days [42, 43, 44]. In a prospective multi-institutional study conducted by Myers E [45] patients were taken for laparoscopic peritoneal lavage with Hinchey 2 or Hinchey 3 diverticulitis [45, 46]. Complete clinical resolution was achieved in all patients except two. One patient required subsequent colonic resection whereas the other required percutaneous drainage for pelvic abscess. Mortality and morbidity rates were 3% and 4%, respectively. After a median follow-up period of 36 months, only two patients were readmitted with acute diverticulitis and subsequently treated successfully with antibiotics. The authors concluded that Laparoscopic lavage drainage can be a good alternative to Hartman procedure for Hinchey 3 perforated diverticulitis. Another prospective study conducted by Liang S et al. [46] found that Laparoscopic lavage drainage has the advantage of shorter operative time and hospital stay, reduced estimated blood loss and better postoperative outcomes as compared to laparoscopic Hartman procedure. Among all patients with complicated diverticulitis (Hinchey 1, 2 and 3), only 2.1% patients undergoing Laparoscopic lavage drainage were converted to open procedure while as 6.4% patients were re-explored for uncontrolled sepsis. Around 50% of the patients who received Laparoscopic lavage drainage underwent subsequent sigmoid resection. Similar favourable results such as low morbidity and mortality rates, better control of sepsis, avoidance of stoma and bowel salvage have been reported in several case series and systematic reviews [37, 47-53].

Agaba et al. [34] reported a favourable outcome after laparoscopic Hartman procedure for Hinchey 3 and 4 diverticulitis in a small case series. To clarify the role of laparoscopy in emergent sigmoidectomy, Mbadiwe et al. [54] analysed data of 11981 patients retrospectively and reported that patients undergoing laparoscopy had lower rates of complications with both resection with primary anastomosis (14% vs 26%, $P < 0.001$) and with Hartmann procedure (30% vs 37%, $P = 0.02$). The mortality rate was less in patients undergoing laparoscopic resection anastomosis as compared to open approach (0.24% vs 0.79%, $P < 0.001$).

In the present era of widespread use of laparoscopy, a well-built RCT is needed to compare laparoscopic resection with primary anastomosis with a two-step laparoscopic HP (sigmoid resection and stoma closure) in perforated complicated diverticulitis, in order to provide a high level of evidence. This will not only help us to know the outcomes of both procedures but would also help us to define the subgroups of patients who will benefit more from each technique.

LAPAROSCOPY IN ELECTIVE SURGERY

Laparoscopy is being increasingly performed for elective surgeries related to complicated diverticulitis. The most common examples are the reversal of Hartman procedure and the sigmoidectomy for chronic complications such as fistula formation, inflammatory stenosis, stricture and phlegmon [55-61].

Several International committees have adopted laparoscopy as the preferred approach for elective sigmoidectomy after acute diverticulitis [1, 23, 24] based on various studies including meta-analysis and RCTs [60-67]. The laparoscopic modality results in less complications, less morbidity, less blood loss, lesser analgesic need, shorter hospital stay and better quality of life compared to open surgery [68, 69].

Laparoscopy was contraindicated previously for the treatment of chronic complications of diverticulitis such as stricture, and fistula due to high risks of bleeding and injury to adjacent organs such as bladder, left ureter, female genital organs [11, 70, 71], because of severe inflammation and distorted anatomy. However, with increased experience in laparoscopy, refinement in technique, and advances in surgical technology, this approach has been widely used as an alternative to open surgery, although its routine use in chronic complications still remains controversial [72].

Colonic fistula is the most commonly reported late complications of diverticular disease in the literature. In a systematic review conducted by Cirocchi R [73] the laparoscopic approach has been reported to be the feasible and safe treatment of colovesical fistulae. But in view of less number of patients and lack of proper methodology, they failed to show superiority of laparoscopy over the open approach. These studies have also not been able to demonstrate the rate of conversion to open method [96]. The outcomes of these studies are difficult to interpret as these studies have included patients with both recurrent uncomplicated and complicated disease. Besides this these studies have also included fistulae due to other aetiologies while interpreting the results. [74-78]. Engledow AH [79], conducted a study over a period of 10 years and included 31 patients in their study. They reported an overall conversion rate of 30% which declined to

10% during the second half of the study period [79]. These findings are consistent with the statement of Abbass et al. [68], who reported similar rates of conversion, morbidity and mortality with laparoscopy irrespective of the presence of colonic fistula. Some studies have demonstrated that severity of disease was a predictor for conversion [80-83], but others could not demonstrate a significant difference [84, 85]. In a multi-centre prospective study of laparoscopic management of diverticulitis, Scheidbach et al. [86] found that complication and conversion rates were initially higher in complicated disease but improved as the surgeon gained experience. In a recent comparative analysis conducted by Lu et al. [3], between laparoscopic versus open anterior resection for recurrent and complicated diverticulitis, significantly shorter operating times, earlier return of bowel function, shorter hospital stay, and a low conversion rate of 3% have been demonstrated. There was no significant difference in morbidity. Over 50% of the laparoscopic group had complicated disease and 21% had a history of multiple previous abdominal surgeries [3]. Overall, recent studies of laparoscopic management of complicated diverticulitis have demonstrated that in the hands of experienced surgeons, morbidity and mortality rates are comparable with open surgery while as the operating times and conversion rates are acceptable [2, 6, 7, 43, 55–58]. Other studies have not used a total laparoscopic approach but have performed resection-facilitated or hand-assisted technique while managing these patients [87-95].

Conclusion

As the use of laparoscopic lavage drainage as a conservative modality of management for complicated perforated diverticulitis has increased, more controversies have emerged about the need for systematic elective sigmoidectomy after the diseased organ has been saved. In a recent systematic review by Cirocchi R, [44], 7% of those patients who underwent Laparoscopic lavage drainage had to be readmitted in hospital. More than 50% of these patients presented with a new episode of diverticulitis, 21% with generalized peritonitis, 10% with colovesical fistula and 7% with undetected colon cancer. At this point of time we don't have enough proof and data, so as to conclude whether LLD can be regarded as a definitive treatment or be considered as a bridge to elective laparoscopic sigmoidectomy [89, 96-103].

REFERENCES

[1] Kohler, L.,Sauerland, S.,Neugebauer, E.(1999). Diagnosis and treatment of diverticular disease: results of a consensus development conference. *The Scientific Committee of the European Association for Endoscopic Surgery. Surg Endosc*, 13(4):430–436. [PubMed] [Google Scholar].

[2] Siddiqui, M.R., Sajid, M.S., Khatri, K., Cheek, E. and Baig, M.K. (2010).Elective open versus laparoscopic sigmoid colectomy for diverticular disease: a meta-analysis with the Sigma trial. *World J Surg*, 34(12):2883–2901. [PubMed] [Google Scholar].

[3] Lu, C.T., Ho, Y.H.(2008).Elective laparoscopic surgical management of recurrent and complicated sigmoid diverticulitis. *Tech Coloproctol*, 12(3):201–206. [PubMed] [Google Scholar].

[4] Li, D., Baxter, N.N., McLeod, R.S., Moineddin, R.,Wilton, A.S. and Nathens, A.B. (2014). Evolving practice patterns in the management of acute colonic diverticulitis: a population-based analysis. *Dis Colon Rectum*, 57:1397–1405. [PubMed] [Google Scholar].

[5] Hinchey, E.J., Schaal, P.G., Richards, G.K.(1978). Treatment of perforated diverticular disease of the colon. *Adv Surg*, 12:85–109. [PubMed] [Google Scholar].

[6] Krukowski, Z.H. and Matheson, N.A.(1984). Emergency surgery for diverticular disease complicated by generalized and faecal peritonitis: A review. *Br J Surg,* 71:921–927. [PubMed] [Google Scholar].

[7] Berry,A.R.,Turner,W.H.,Mortensen,N.J. and Kettlewell,M.G. (1989).Emergency surgery for complicated diverticular disease. A five-year experience. *Dis Colon Rectum,* 32:849–854. [PubMed] [Google Scholar].

[8] Salem, L., Anaya, D.A. and Flum, D.R. (2005). Temporal changes in the management of diverticulitis. *J Surg Res*, 124;318–323. [PubMed] [Google Scholar].

[9] Kronborg, O.(1993). Treatment of perforated sigmoid diverticulitis: a prospective randomized trial. *Br J Surg,* 80:505–507. [PubMed] [Google Scholar].

[10] Khan, A.L., Ah-See, A.K., Crofts, T.J., Heys, S.D and Eremin, O. (1995). Surgical management of the septic complications of diverticular disease. *Ann R Coll Surg Engl,* 77: 16–20. [PMC free article] [PubMed] [Google Scholar].

[11] Köhler, L., Sauerland, S.,and Neugebauer, E. (1999). Diagnosis and treatment of diverticular disease: Results of a consensus development conference. The Scientific Committee of the European Association for Endoscopic Surgery. *Surg Endosc,* 13:430–436. [PubMed] [Google Scholar].

[12] Stollman, N.H. and Raskin, J.B.(1999). Diagnosis and management of diverticular disease of the colon in adults. Ad Hoc Practice Parameters Committee of the American College of Gastroenterology. *Am J Gastroenterol,* 94: 3110–3121. [PubMed] [Google Scholar].

[13] Wong, W.D., Wexner, S.D., Lowry, A., Vernava, A., Burnstein, M., Denstman, F., Fazio, V.,Kerner, B., Moore, R. and Oliver, G. (2000). Practice parameters for the treatment of sigmoid diverticulitis--supporting documentation. The Standards Task Force. The American Society of Colon and Rectal Surgeons. *Dis Colon Rectum*,43:290–297. [PubMed] [Google Scholar].

[14] Salem, L.,Anaya, D.A., Roberts, K.E. and Flum, D.R.(2005). Hartmann's colectomy and reversal in diverticulitis: A population-level assessment. *Dis Colon Rectum*, 48:988–995. [PubMed] [Google Scholar].

[15] Seah, D.W., Ibrahim, S. and Tay, K.H.(2005). Hartmann procedure: is it still relevant today? *ANZ J Surg,* 75, 436–440. [PubMed] [Google Scholar].

[16] Maggard,M.A., Zingmond, D., O'Connell, J.B. and Ko, C.Y. (2004). What proportion of patients with an ostomy (for diverticulitis) get reversed? *Am Surg,* 70;928–931. [PubMed] [Google Scholar].

[17] Chapman, J; Davies, M; Wolff, B; Dozois, E; Tessier, D; Harrington, J; Larson, D.(2005). Complicated diverticulitis: is it time to rethink the rules? *Ann Surg,* 242 :576–581, discussion 581-583 [PMC free article] [PubMed] [Google Scholar].

[18] Ince, M., Stocchi, L., Khomvilai, S., Kwon, D.S., Hammel, J.P and Kiran, R.P.(2012). Morbidity and mortality of the Hartmann procedure for diverticular disease over 18 years in a single institution. *Colorectal Dis,* 14: e492–e498. [PubMed] [Google Scholar].

[19] Schwenk, W., Haase, O., Neudecker, J. and Müller, J.M.(2005). Short term benefits for laparoscopic colorectal resection. *Cochrane Database Syst Rev*. (3):CD003145. [PubMed] [Google Scholar].

[20] Braga, M., Vignali, A., Gianotti, L., Zuliani, W., Radaelli, G., Gruarin, P., Dellabona, P. and Di, Carlo, V.(2002). Laparoscopic versus open colorectal surgery: a randomized trial on short-term outcome. *Ann Surg,* 236:759–766, disscussion 767. [PMC free article] [PubMed] [Google Scholar].

[21] Delaney, C.P., Chang, E., Senagore, AJ. and Broder, M.(2008). Clinical outcomes and resource utilization associated with laparoscopic and open colectomy using a large national database. *Ann Surg,* 247: 819–824. [PubMed] [Google Scholar].

[22] Forgione, A., Leroy, J., Cahill, RA., Bailey, C., Simone, M., Mutter, D and Marescaux, J.(2009). Prospective evaluation of functional outcome after laparoscopic sigmoid colectomy. *Ann Surg,* 249; 218–224. [PubMed] [Google Scholar].

[23] Rafferty, J.,Shellito, P., Hyman, N.H. and Buie, W.D. (2006). Practice parameters for sigmoid diverticulitis. *Dis Colon Rectum,* 49:939–944. [PubMed] [Google Scholar].

[24] Fozard, J.B., Armitage, N.C., Schofield, J.B. and Jones, O.M. (2011).ACPGBI position statement on elective resection for diverticulitis. *Colorectal Dis,* 13(3); 1–11. [PubMed] [Google Scholar].

[25] Sauerland, S., Agresta, F., Bergamaschi, R., Borzellino, G;., Budzynski, A., Champault, G., Fingerhut, A., Isla, A., Johansson, M.and Lundorff, P. (2006). Laparoscopy for abdominal emergencies: evidence-based guidelines of the European Association for Endoscopic Surgery. *Surg Endosc*, 20, 14–29. [PubMed] [Google Scholar].

[26] Turley, R.S., Barbas, A.S., Lidsky, M.E., Mantyh, C.R., Migaly, J.and Scarborough, J.E.(2013). Laparoscopic versus open Hartmann procedure for the emergency treatment of diverticulitis: a propensity-matched analysis. *Dis Colon Rectum,* 56: 72–82. [PMC free article] [PubMed] [Google Scholar].

[27] Vermeulen, J. and Lange, J.F.(2010). Treatment of perforated diverticulitis with generalized peritonitis: Past, present, and future. *World J Surg,* 34:587–593. [PMC free article] [PubMed] [Google Scholar].

[28] Stocchi, L.(2010).Current indications and role of surgery in the management of sigmoid diverticulitis. *World J Gastroenterol*, 16: 804–817. [PMC free article] [PubMed] [Google Scholar].

[29] Stulberg, J.J., Champagne, B.J., Fan, Z., Horan, M., Obias, V., Marderstein, E., Reynolds, H. and Delaney, C.P.(2009). Emergency laparoscopic colectomy: does it measure up to open? *Am J Surg,* 197: 296–301. [PMC free article] [PubMed] [Google Scholar].

[30] Chand, M., Siddiqui, M.R., Gupta, A., Rasheed, S., Tekkis, P., Parvaiz, A., Mirnezami, A.H. and Qureshi, T.(2014). Systematic review of emergent laparoscopic colorectal surgery for benign and malignant disease. *World J Gastroenterol*, 20: 16956–16963. [PMC free article] [PubMed] [Google Scholar].

[31] Gaertner, W.B., Kwaan, M.R., Madoff, R.D.,Willis, D., Belzer, G.E., Rothenberger, D.A.and Melton, G.B. (2013). The evolving role of laparoscopy in colonic diverticular disease: a systematic review. *World J Surg,* 37 :629–638. [PubMed] [Google Scholar].

[32] Anderson, C.A., Fowler, D.L., White, S. and Wintz, N. (1993). Laparoscopic colostomy closure. *Surg Laparosc Endosc,* 3; 69–72. [PubMed] [Google Scholar].

[33] Chouillard, E., Maggiori, L., Ata, T., Jarbaoui, S., Rivkine, E., Benhaim, L., Ghiles, E., Etienne, JC. and Fingerhut, A. (2007). Laparoscopic two-stage left colonic resection for patients with peritonitis caused by acute diverticulitis. *Dis Colon Rectum,* 50:1157–1163. [PubMed] [Google Scholar].

[34] Agaba, E.A., Zaidi, R.M., Ramzy, P., Aftab, M., Rubach, E., Gecelter, G., Ravikumar, TS. and DeNoto, G.(2009). Laparoscopic Hartmann's procedure: a viable option for treatment of acutely perforated diverticultis. *Surg Endosc,* 23: 1483–1486. [PubMed] [Google Scholar].

[35] Regenbogen, S.E., Hardiman, K.M., Hendren, S. and Morris, A.M. (2014). Surgery for diverticulitis in the 21st century: a systematic review. *JAMA Surg,* 149:292–303. [PubMed] [Google Scholar].

[36] Bretagnol, F., Pautrat, K., Mor, C., Benchellal, Z., Huten, N. and de, Calan, L.(2008). Emergency laparoscopic management of perforated sigmoid diverticulitis: a promising alternative to more radical procedures. *J Am Coll Surg,* 206: 654–657. [PubMed] [Google Scholar].

[37] Alamili, M., Gögenur, I. and Rosenberg, J.(2009). Acute complicated diverticulitis managed by laparoscopic lavage. *Dis Colon Rectum,* 52; 1345–1349. [PubMed] [Google Scholar].

[38] Wieghard, N., Geltzeiler, C.B. and Tsikitis, V.L.(2015). Trends in the surgical management of diverticulitis. *Ann Gastroenterol,* 28: 25–30. [PMC free article] [PubMed] [Google Scholar].

[39] Moore, FA., Catena, F., Moore, E.E, Leppaniemi, A., Peitzmann, A.B.(2013). Position paper: management of perforated sigmoid diverticulitis. *World J Emerg Surg,* 8: 55. [PMC free article] [PubMed] [Google Scholar].

[40] Letarte, F., Hallet, J., Drolet, S., Charles, A Grégoire, R., Bouchard, A., Gagné, J.P., Thibault, C. and Bouchard, P. (2013). Laparoscopic emergency surgery for diverticular disease that failed medical treatment: a valuable option? Results of a retrospective comparative cohort study. *Dis Colon Rectum,* 56 :1395–1402. [PubMed] [Google Scholar].

[41] Letarte, F., Hallet, J., Drolet, S., Boulanger-Gobeil, C., Bouchard, A., Grégoire, R.C., Gagné, J.P., Thibault, C. and Bouchard, P. (2015). Laparoscopic versus open colonic resection for complicated diverticular disease in the emergency setting: a safe choice? A retrospective comparative cohort study. *Am J Surg,* 209 : 992–998. [PubMed] [Google Scholar].

[42] O'Sullivan, G.C., Murphy, D., O'Brien, M.G. and Ireland, A. (1996). Laparoscopic management of generalized peritonitis due to perforated colonic diverticula. *Am J Surg,* 171; 432–434. [PubMed] [Google Scholar].

[43] Rizk, N. and Champault, G.(1996). Laparoscopic treatment in two operative stages of perforated sigmoid diverticulitis: 2 cases. *Ann Chir,* 50: 283. [PubMed] [Google Scholar].

[44] Cirocchi, R., Trastulli, S., Vettoretto, N., Milani, D., Cavaliere, D., Renzi, C., Adamenko, O., Desiderio, J., Burattini, M.F and Parisi, A et al. (2015). Laparoscopic peritoneal lavage: a definitive treatment for diverticular peritonitis or a "bridge" to elective laparoscopic sigmoidectomy? *A systematic review. Medicine (Baltimore),* 94; e334. [PMC free article] [PubMed] [Google Scholar].

[45] Myers, E., Hurley, M., O'Sullivan, G.C., Kavanagh, D., Wilson, I., Winter, D.C. (2008). Laparoscopic peritoneal lavage for generalized peritonitis due to perforated diverticulitis. *Br J Surg,* 95:97–101. [PubMed] [Google Scholar].

[46] Liang, S., Russek, K. and Franklin, M.E.(2012). Damage control strategy for the management of perforated diverticulitis with generalized peritonitis: laparoscopic lavage and drainage vs. laparoscopic Hartmann's procedure. *Surg Endosc,* 26; 2835–2842. [PubMed] [Google Scholar].

[47] Toorenvliet, B.R., Swank, H., Schoones, J.W., Hamming, J.F., Bemelman, W.A. (2010). Laparoscopic peritoneal lavage for perforated colonic diverticulitis: a systematic review. *Colorectal Dis,* 12; 862–867. [PubMed] [Google Scholar].

[48] Rogers, A.C., Collins, D., O'Sullivan, G.C.and Winter, D.C. (2012). Laparoscopic lavage for perforated diverticulitis: A population

analysis. *Dis Colon Rectum*, 55 : 932–938. [PubMed] [Google Scholar].

[49] White, S.I., Frenkiel, B. and Martin, P.J. (2010). A ten-year audit of perforated sigmoid diverticulitis: Highlighting the outcomes of laparoscopic lavage. *Dis Colon Rectum,* 53:1537–1541. [PubMed] [Google Scholar].

[50] Edeiken, S.M., Maxwell, R.A., Dart, B.W. and Mejia, V.A. (2013). Preliminary experience with laparoscopic peritoneal lavage for complicated diverticulitis: A new algorithm for treatment? *Am Surg,* 79: 819–825. [PubMed] [Google Scholar].

[51] McDermott, F.D., Collins, D., Heeney, A. and Winter, D.C. (2014). Minimally invasive and surgical management strategies tailored to the severity of acute diverticulitis. *Br J Surg,* 101: e90–e99. [PubMed] [Google Scholar].

[52] Afshar, S. and Kurer, MA.(2012). Laparoscopic peritoneal lavage for perforated sigmoid diverticulitis. *Colorectal Dis*, 14; 135–142. [PubMed] [Google Scholar]

[53] Rossi, G.L., Mentz, R., Bertone, S.,Ojea, Quintana, G., Bilbao, S., Im, V.M. and Vaccaro, C.A.(2014). Laparoscopic peritoneal lavage for Hinchey III diverticulitis: Is it as effective as it is applicable? *Dis Colon Rectum,* 57:1384–1390. [PubMed].

[54] Mbadiwe, T., Obirieze, AC., Cornwell, EE., Turner, P., and Fullum, T.M.(2013). Surgical management of complicated diverticulitis: a comparison of the laparoscopic and open approaches. *J Am Coll Surg,* 216: 782–788, discussion 788-790. [PubMed] [Google Scholar].

[55] Feingold, D., Steele, S.R., Lee, S., Kaiser, A., Boushey, R., Buie, WD. and Rafferty, J.F.(2014). Practice parameters for the treatment of sigmoid diverticulitis. *Dis Colon Rectum.*,57: 284–294. [PubMed] [Google Scholar].

[56] Angenete, E., Thornell, A., Burcharth, J., Pommergaard, HC., Skullman, S., Bisgaard, T., Jess, P., Läckberg, Z., Matthiessen, P., Heath, J., et al. (2016). Laparoscopic Lavage Is Feasible and Safe for the Treatment of Perforated Diverticulitis With Purulent Peritonitis: The First Results From the Randomized Controlled Trial DILALA.

Ann Surg, 263: 117–122. [PMC free article] [PubMed] [Google Scholar].

[57] Vennix, S., Musters, G.D., Mulder, I.M., Swank, H.A., Consten, E.C., Belgers, E.H., Van, Geloven, A.A., Gerhards, M..F., Govaert, M..J. and Van, Grevenstein, W.M. et al. (2015). Laparoscopic peritoneal lavage or sigmoidectomy for perforated diverticulitis with purulent peritonitis: a multicentre, parallel-group, randomised, open-label trial. *Lancet*, 386:1269–1277. [PubMed] [Google Scholar].

[58] Swank, H.A., Mulder, I.M., Hoofwijk, A.G., Nienhuijs, S.W., Lange, J.F. and Bemelman, WA.(2013). Early experience with laparoscopic lavage for perforated diverticulitis. *Br J Surg*, 100 :704–710. [PubMed] [Google Scholar].

[59] Radé, F., Bretagnol, F.,Auguste, M., Di Guisto, C., Huten, N. and de Calan, L. (2014). Determinants of outcome following laparoscopic peritoneal lavage for perforated diverticulitis. *Br J Surg,* 101 : 1602–166, discussion 1606. [PubMed] [Google Scholar].

[60] Bethesda, M.D. Laparoscopic Lavage for Acute Non-Faeculant Diverticulitis. In: *Clinical Trials.gov* [Internet]. National Library of Medicine (US), St Vincent's University Hospital, Ireland LapLAND Available from: https://clinicaltrials.gov/ct2/show/{"type": "clinical-trial","attrs": {"text": "NCT01019239","term_id": "NCT01019239"}}NCT01019239 NLM Identifier: {"type", "clinical-trial","attrs": {"text": "NCT01019239","term_id":"NCT01019239"}} NCT01019239.

[61] Bethesda,M.D. Diverticulitis Trial (SCANDIV). In: *Clinical Trials.gov* [Internet]. Bethesda (MD): National Library of Medicine (US) University Hospital, Akershus Scandinavian Available from: https://clinicaltrials.gov/ct2/show/{"type": "clinical-trial", "attrs": {"text": "NCT01047462","term_id", "NCT01047462"}} NCT01047462 NLM Identifier: {"type": "clinical-trial", "attrs": {"text": "NCT01047462","term_id":"NCT01047462"}} NCT01047462.

[62] Mutter, D., Bouras, G., Forgione, A., Vix, M., Leroy, J., and Marescaux, J. (2006). Two-stage totally minimally invasive approach

for acute complicated diverticulitis. *Colorectal Dis*. 8: 501–505. [PubMed] [Google Scholar].

[63] Salem, L. and Flum, D.R. (2004). Primary anastomosis or Hartmann's procedure for patients with diverticular peritonitis? A systematic review. *Dis Colon Rectum.* 47: 1953–1964. [PubMed] [Google Scholar].

[64] Schilling, M.K., Maurer, C.A., Kollmar, O. and Büchler, M.W. (2001). Primary vs. secondary anastomosis after sigmoid colon resection for perforated diverticulitis (Hinchey Stage III and IV): A prospective outcome and cost analysis. *Dis Colon Rectum, 44*; 699–703, discussion 703-5. [PubMed] [Google Scholar].

[65] Gooszen, A.W., Gooszen, H.G., Veerman, W., Van Dongen, V.M., Hermans, J., Klien, Kranenbarg, E. and Tollenaar, R.A.(2001). Operative treatment of acute complications of diverticular disease: primary or secondary anastomosis after sigmoid resection. *Eur J Surg.*167 : 35–39. [PubMed] [Google Scholar].

[66] Vermeulen, J., Coene, P.P., Van, Hout, N.M., van, der, Harst, E., Gosselink, M.P., Mannaerts, G.H., Weidema, W.F; and Lange, J.F.(2009).Restoration of bowel continuity after surgery for acute perforated diverticulitis: should Hartmann's procedure be considered a one-stage procedure? *Colorectal Dis*, 11 : 619–624. [PubMed] [Google Scholar].

[67] Toro, A., Mannino, M., Reale, G., Cappello, G. and Di, Carlo, I. (2012). Primary anastomosis vs Hartmann procedure in acute complicated diverticulitis. Evolution over the last twenty years. *Chirurgia (Bucur),*107 : 598–604. [PubMed] [Google Scholar].

[68] Abbas, S.(2007). Resection and primary anastomosis in acute complicated diverticulitis, a systematic review of the literature. *Int J Colorectal Dis,* 22 : 351–357. [PubMed] [Google Scholar].

[69] Constantinides, V.A., Tekkis, P.P., Athanasiou, T., Aziz, O., Purkayastha, S., Remzi, FH., Fazio, VW., Aydin, N., Darzi, A. and Senapati, A. (2006). Primary resection with anastomosis vs. Hartmann's procedure in nonelective surgery for acute colonic

diverticulitis: a systematic review. *Dis Colon Rectum*. 49 : 966–981. [PubMed] [Google Scholar].

[70] Constantinides, V.A., Heriot, A., Remzi, F., Darzi, A., Senapati, A., Fazio, VW. and Tekkis, P.P. (2007). Operative strategies for diverticular peritonitis: a decision analysis between primary resection and anastomosis versus Hartmann's procedures. *Ann Surg*, 245 : 94–103. [PMC free article] [PubMed] [Google Scholar].

[71] Zorcolo, L., Covotta, L., Carlomagno, N. and Bartolo, D.C.(2003). Safety of primary anastomosis in emergency colo-rectal surgery. *Colorectal Dis,* 5 : 262–269. [PubMed] [Google Scholar].

[72] Breitenstein, S., Kraus, A., Hahnloser, D., Decurtins, M., Clavien, PA. and Demartines, N.(2007). Emergency left colon resection for acute perforation: primary anastomosis or Hartmann's procedure? A case-matched control study. *World J Surg,* 31 : 2117–2124. [PubMed] [Google Scholar].

[73] Alizai, P. H., Schulze-Hagen, M., Klink, C.D; Ulmer, F., Roeth, A. A., Neumann, U.P., Jansen, M., Rosch, R. (2013). Primary anastomosis with a defunctioning stoma versus Hartmann's procedure for perforated diverticulitis--a comparison of stoma reversal rates. *Int J Colorectal Dis*, 28 : 1681–1688. [PubMed] [Google Scholar].

[74] Joo, J.S., Agachan, F., Wexner, S.D.(1997). Laparoscopic surgery for lower gastrointestinal fistulas. *Surg Endosc,* 11 (2) :116–118. [PubMed] [Google Scholar].

[75] Poulin, E.C., Schlachta, C.M., Mamazza, J. and Seshadri, P.A. (2000). Should enteric fistulas from Crohn's disease or diverticulitis be treated laparoscopically or by open surgery? *Dis Colon Rectum,* 43(5) : 621–627. [PubMed] [Google Scholar].

[76] Regan, J.P and Salky, B.A.(2004). Laparoscopic treatment of enteric fistulas. *Surg Endosc*, 18 (2) : 252–254. [PubMed] (Google Scholar).

[77] Moorthy, K., Shaul, T. and Foley, R.J.(2004). The laparoscopic management of benign bowel fistulas. *JSLS*, 8(4): 356–358. [PMC free article] [PubMed] [Google Scholar].

[78] Pokala, N., Delaney, C.P., Brady, K.M., Senagore, A. .J.(2005). Elective laparoscopic surgery for benign internal enteric fistulas: a

review of 43 cases. *Surg Endosc*, 19(2) :222–225. [PubMed] [Google Scholar].

[79] Engledow, A.H., Pakzad, F., Ward, N.J., Arulampalam, T. and Motson, R.W. (2007). Laparoscopic resection of diverticular fistulae: a 10-year experience. *Colorectal Dis*, 9 : 632–634. [PubMed] [Google Scholar].

[80] Sher, M.E., Agachan, F., Bortul, M., Nogueras, J.J., Weiss, E.G. and Wexner, S.D.(1997). Laparoscopic surgery for diverticulitis. *Surg Endosc*, 11(3), 264–267. [PubMed] [Google Scholar].

[81] Garrett, K.A., Champagne, B.J.,Valerian, B.T.,Peterson, D. and Lee, E.C. (2008). A single training center's experience with 200 consecutive cases of diverticulitis: can all patients be approached laparoscopically? *Surg Endosc*, 22(11) : 2503–2508. [PubMed] [Google Scholar].

[82] Reissfelder, C., Buhr, H.J. and Ritz, J.P.(2006) Can laparoscopically assisted sigmoid resection provide uncomplicated management even in cases of complicated diverticulitis? *Surg Endosc*, 20(7) : 1055–1059. [PubMed] [Google Scholar].

[83] Martel, G ., Bouchard, A ., Soto, C.M., Poulin, E.C., Mamazza, J.(2010). Boushey, R.P. Laparoscopic colectomy for complex diverticular disease: a justifiable choice? *Surg Endosc*, 24(9) : 2273–2280. [PubMed] [Google Scholar].

[84] Stevenson, A.R., Stitz, RW., Lumley, JW. and Fielding, GA.(1998). Laparoscopic assisted anterior resection for diverticular disease: follow-up of 100 consecutive patients. *Ann Surg*, 227(3) : 335–342. [PMC free article] [PubMed] [Google Scholar] 84.

[85] Hassan, I., Cima, R.R., Larson, D.W., Dozois, E.J., Byrne, M.M. and Larson, DR, et al.(2007). The impact of uncomplicated and complicated diverticulitis on laparoscopic surgery conversion rates and patient outcomes. *Surg Endosc*, 21(10) : 1690–1694. [PubMed] [Google Scholar] 85.

[86] Scheidbach, H., Schneider, C., Rose, J., Konradt, J., Gross, E. and Barlehner, E; et al.(2004). Laparoscopic approach to treatment of sigmoid diverticulitis: changes in the spectrum of indications and

results of a prospective, multicenter study on 1,545 patients. *Dis Colon Rectum*, 47(11) : 1883–1888. [PubMed] [Google Scholar].

[87] Lee, S.W., Yoo, J., Dujovny, N., Sonoda, T. and Milsom, J.W. (2006). Laparoscopic vs. hand-assisted laparoscopic sigmoidectomy for diverticulitis. *Dis Colon Rectum*, 49(4) : 464–469. [PubMed] [Google Scholar].

[88] Pendlimari, R., Touzios, J.G., Azodo, A., Chua, H.K., Dozois, E.J; and Cima, R.R; et al.(2011). Short-term outcomes after elective minimally invasive colectomy for diverticulitis. *Br J Surg*, 98(3) : 431–435. [PubMed] [Google Scholar].

[89] Eijsbouts, QA., de Haan, J., Berends, F., Sietses, C. and Cuesta, M.A. (2000). Laparoscopic elective treatment of diverticular disease: a comparison between laparoscopic-assisted and resection-facilitated techniques. *Surg Endosc*, 14(8):726–730. [PubMed] [Google Scholar].

[90] Gervaz, P., Inan, I., Perneger, T., Schiffer, E. and Morel, P. (2010). A prospective, randomized, single-blind comparison of laparoscopic versus open sigmoid colectomy for diverticulitis. *Ann Surg*, 252 : 3–8. [PubMed] [Google Scholar].

[91] Vargas, H.D., Ramirez, R.T., Hoffman, G.C., Hubbard, G.W., Gould, R.J., Wohlgemuth, S.D., Ruffin, W.K., Hatter, J.E. and Kolm, P. (2000). Defining the role of laparoscopic-assisted sigmoid colectomy for diverticulitis. *Dis Colon Rectum*, 43 : 1726–1731. [PubMed] [Google Scholar].

[92] Collins, D. and Winter, D. C.(2014). Laparoscopy in diverticular disease: Controversies. *Best Pract Res Clin Gastroenterol*, 28: 175–182. [PubMed] [Google Scholar].

[93] Le, Moine, M. C; Fabre, J. M; Vacher, C; Navarro, F; Picot, M. C; and Domergue, J.(2003). Factors and consequences of conversion in laparoscopic sigmoidectomy for diverticular disease. *Br J Surg*, 90 : 232–236. [PubMed] [Google Scholar].

[94] De, Magistris, L., Azagra, J.S., Goergen, M., De, Blasi, V., Arru, L.and Facy, O.(2013). Laparoscopic sigmoidectomy in moderate and severe diverticulitis: analysis of short-term outcomes in a continuous

series of 121 patients. *Surg Endosc*, 27:1766–1771. [PubMed] [Google Scholar].

[95] Pendlimari, R., Touzios, J.G., Azodo, I.A., Chua, H.K., Dozois, E.J., Cima, R.R. and Larson, D.W.(2011). Short-term outcomes after elective minimally invasive colectomy for diverticulitis. *Br J Surg*, 98 : 431–435. [PubMed] [Google Scholar].

[96] Cirocchi, R., Cochetti, G., Randolph, J., Listorti, C., Castellani, E., Renzi, C., Mearini, E., and Fingerhut, A.(2014). Laparoscopic treatment of colovesical fistulas due to complicated colonic diverticular disease: a systematic review. *Tech Coloproctol*, 18: 873–885. [PubMed] [Google Scholar] (73)

[97] Laurent, S.R., Detroz, B., Detry, O., Degauque, C., Honoré, P. and Meurisse, M.(2005). Laparoscopic sigmoidectomy for fistulized diverticulitis. *Dis Colon Rectum*, 48 : 148–152. [PubMed] [Google Scholar].

[98] Engledow, A.H., Pakzad, F., Ward, N.J., Arulampalam, T. and Motson, R.W.(2007). Laparoscopic resection of diverticular fistulae: a 10-year experience. *Colorectal Dis*, 9: 632–634. [PubMed] [Google Scholar] 79.

[99] Abbass, M.A ., Tsay, A.T. and Abbas, M.A. (2013). Laparoscopic resection of chronic sigmoid diverticulitis with fistula. *JSLS*, 17 :636–640. [PMC free article] [PubMed] [Google Scholar].

[100] Sorrentino, M., Brizzolari, M., Scarpa, E., Malisan, D., Bruschi, F., Bertozzi, S., Bernardi, S. and Petri, R. (2015). Laparoscopic peritoneal lavage for perforated colonic diverticulitis: a definitive treatment? Retrospective analysis of 63 cases. *Tech Coloproctol*, 19 :105–110. [PubMed] [Google Scholar].

[101] Marusch, F., Gastinger, I., Schneider, C., Scheidbach, H., Konradt, J. and Bruch, H.P., et al. (2001). Experience as a factor influencing the indications for laparoscopic colorectal surgery and the results. *Surg Endosc*, 15(2) : 116–120. [PubMed] [Google Scholar].

[102] Vermeulen, J. and Lange, J.F. (2010) Treatment of perforated diverticulitis with generalized peritonitis: past, present, and future. *World J Surg,* 34(3): 587-93. [PubMed].

[103] Gaertner, W.B., Kwaan, M.R., Madoff, R.D., Willis, D., Belzer, G.E., Rothenberger, D.A. and Melton, G.B.(2013). Review; The evolving role of laparoscopy in colonic diverticular disease: a systematic review. *World J Surg*, 37(3) : 629-38. [PubMed].

In: Diverticulitis: Diagnosis and Treatment ISBN: 978-1-53618-081-7
Editors: Shams-ul-Bari et al.

Chapter 8

RECURRENT ACUTE DIVERTICULITIS

Ajaz Ahmad Rather*
Department of Surgery. SKIMS Medical College,
Bemina Srinagar, Kashmir

ABSTRACT

Acute diverticulitis is an inflammation due to a small perforation of a sac like protrusion of the colonic wall. Recurrent attacks of acute diverticulitis are seen in 20-35% of patients after first attack. Though the recurrence of diverticulitis is common, yet there is no tool to assess which patients are prone to get the recurrent attacks and who will have complicated recurrence. The prevalence of diverticulitis has increased at the start of twentieth century which can be attributed to the several reasons. There has been an increase in the life expectancy throughout the globe; more number of cases have been detected. It has been found that in western countries about 50% of individuals develop diverticulosis. About 5-10% of the patients develop it by the age of 40 years, with an alarming increase up to 65% by the age of 80 years. Secondly, westernization of dietary habits such as shift of food habits from high fibre to low fibre diets, especially high intake of red meat, consumption of refined sugars and milled floor, low intake of fruits, cereals and vegetables. This relation of dietary fibre

---

* Corresponding Author's Email: drajazrather@gmail.com.

has been described by Painter & Burkit based on their study in 1970's in Sub Saharan Africa.

It is an established fact that lack of fibre in the diet leads to constipation. Straining due to constipation leads to segmentation and herniation of mucosa because of high pressure, especially in the sigmoid colon. It has been found that the herniation of mucosa occurs at the weaker points in the gut well,where the blood vessels (vasa recta) penetrate to reach mucosa and sub mucosa.

INTRODUCTION

Acute diverticulitis is an inflammation due to a small perforation of a sac like protrusion of the colonic wall. Although recurrent attacks of acute diverticulitis have been reported in 20-35% of patients but there is no tool to assess which patients are prone to get the recurrent attacks and who will have complicated recurrence. The prevalence of diverticulitis has increased at the start of twentieth century due to several reasons. Increase in the life expectancy throughout the globe with detection of more number of cases could be one reason. It has been found that in western countries about 50% of individuals develop diverticulosis. Out of them 5-10% develop diverticulosis by the age of 40 years with an alarming increase up to 65% by the age of 80 years [1].

Westernization of dietary habits is the main factor involved in the etiopathogenesis of diverticulitis, which includes change of dietary habits from high fibre to low fibre diets, especially high intake of red meat, consumption of refined sugars and milled floor along with low intake of fruits, cereals and vegetables. This relation of dietary fibre has been described by Painter & Burkit based on their study in 1970's in Sub Saharan Africa [2]. It is a well-known fact that lack of fibre in the diet leads to constipation and straining, which leads to segmentation and herniation of mucosa due to high pressure, especially in the sigmoid colon. Herniation of mucosa occurs at the weaker points in the gut well where the blood vessels (vasa recta breva) penetrate to reach mucosa and sub mucosa. `In western population, sigmoid colon is involved in up to 90- 95%, in contrast to the Asian population where right side disease is more common [3].

Plain X-ray abdomen in supine and upright left lateral decubitus position may be an initial investigation which may show free gas in abdomen if there is any perforation of diverticulum. It may also depict localized ileus because of inflammation or features of gut obstruction.

Contrast enhanced CT Abdomen is a preferred initial investigation for evaluation of patients with diverticulitis. Contrast may be given intravenously, orally or rectally. In case of diverticulitis stranding of pericolic fat may be seen. Hinchey & co-workers described four stages of the disease. Stage I in which there is a pericolic abscess confined to the mesentery of colon, stage II in which there is pelvic abscess resulting from extension of pericolic abscess, stage III characterised by purulent peritonitis and stage IV characterised by feculent peritonitis.

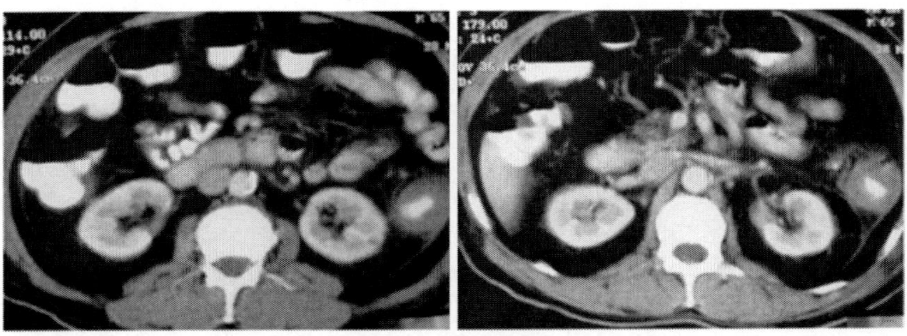

Figure 1. CT picture showing (axial view) Post diverticulitis pericolic collection.

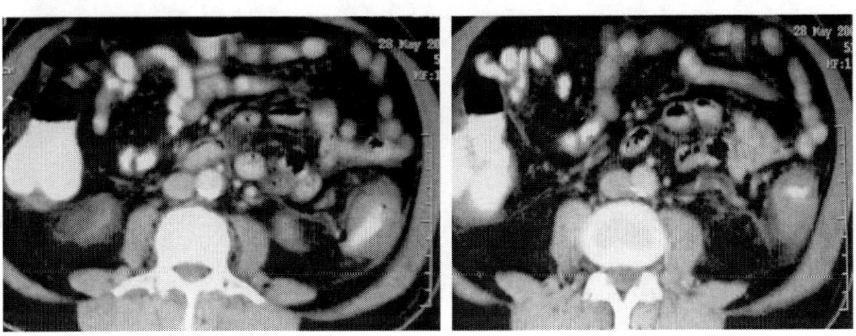

Figure 2. CT picture showing Post diverticulitis pericolic collection.

Contrast study may be also be helpful in identifying fistulas most commonly colo-vaginal or colo-enteric. CT plays an important role in diagnosing and staging of acute diverticulitis and has also valuable role in patients with diverticular abscess where thickening of colonic wall and presence of air in abscess may be detected (Figures 1 & 2).

Barium Enema

It is contraindicated in initial stages of acute diverticulitis as barium may leak into peritoneal cavity. However, water soluble contrast used under low pressure is safe. Barium enema (Figures 3, 4) can be done after a week when the acute inflammation has subsided. Some people prefer barium enema as it gives us idea about the extent of diverticulosis in the colon and can also assess the length of stricture in colon; however it seems to have a limited role at present.

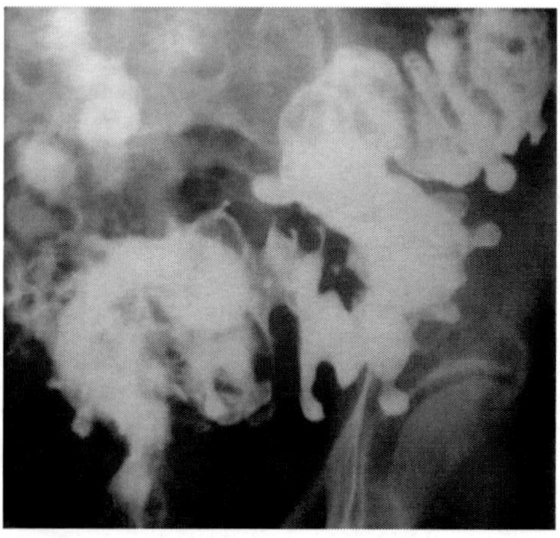

Figure 3. Barium contrast showing diverticuli in colon.

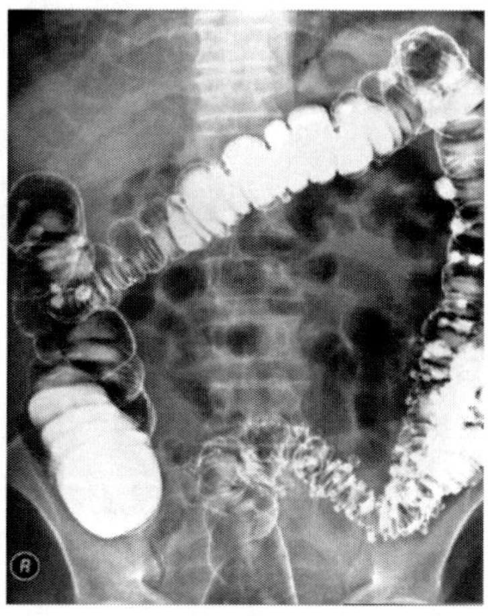

Figure 4. Barium contrast showing diverticuli in colon.

Recurrent Diverticulitis

Recurrent diverticulitis usually occurs in a patient who has been medically managed for an attack of diverticulitis. Rarely it may occur in a patient who has undergone surgery for sigmoid diverticulosis. What causes the increase in incidence of a nonsurgicaly managed patient is not known as there is an insufficient material in literature to determine the risk factors. It has been found by Hupfield et al. [4] that younger people less than 50 years of age and those who had a diverticular abscess formation are at higher risk of not only recurrence (27 vs. 17%) but also have got higher chances of undergoing surgery (colectomy /colostomy (7.5% vs. 5%) [4]. Since the incidence of diverticulosis has increased so one can logically expect an increase in the frequency of recurrent acute diverticulitis.

Risk Factors for Recurrent Diverticulitis

The risk of developing recurrent attacks of diverticulitis after recovery from an attack of diverticulitis has been found to be around 30-36%. This means that a majority of the patients have no further attack of diverticulitis. It has been noted that a patient with long segment diverticulitis (>5 cms) on CT scan and those with family history of diverticulosis are at an increased risk of developing subsequent attacks.

The clinical course of diverticulitis appears to be determined by first attack. Those patients who present with uncomplicated diverticulitis do not usually progress to subsequent attacks of complicated diverticulitis. The risk of having subsequent attacks of complicated diverticulitis after recovery from an attack of uncomplicated diverticulitis has been shown by many studies to be less than 5%.

El Sayed et al. [5] found a recurrence rate of 11.2% over a follow up period of 4 years, in a study involving 65000 patients who were managed non-operatively. Risk factors for readmission and emergency surgery were female sex, young age, smoking, obesity and complicated initial disease. Emergency and elective colectomy rates were 0.9% and 0.75% in this series.

Ville Sallinen et al. [6] conducted a study involving 512 patients and proposed a simple risk score on the basis of which patients have been divided into low-risk and high-risk patient populations to predict recurrence of complicated diverticulitis. The risk score consists of 3 simple bed-side parameters which include history of diverticulitis, history of abscess and corticosteroid medication.

Patients who have a history of three or more attacks of diverticulitis are at great risk for developing attacks of uncomplicated recurrence, while at the same time it does not increase the risk for complicated recurrence. Ville Sallinen et al. [6] have proposed that if several attacks of recurrent diverticulitis is used as the only indication for prophylactic sigmoid resection, the operation will lower risk of uncomplicated recurrence rate, but might not be effective in preventing complicated recurrence. They have reported an overall 5-year recurrence of 39% and complicated recurrence rate of 5% which were similar to those reported by others (36% and 3.9%) [7, 8]. Thus, complicated recurrence rate is low, and careful patient selection is needed to prevent complicated recurrence.

However this study had some limitations. Firstly, this was a single-centre based retrospective Cohort study. Secondly, follow-up was done by examining the health records of patients maintained in medical record sections of the hospitals and patients were not contacted. This may lead to underestimation of the recurrence rate as many patients do not report to hospital for follow up. Thirdly, 23% of patients underwent an elective sigmoid resection in the follow-up. Since sigmoid resection prevents majority of recurrences, it will have a major impact on the recurrence rates. Another limitations was that only a limited number of patients developed a complicated recurrence over a follow-up period of 5 years (26 out of 512 patients), which merely shows that complicated recurrence is rare. They concluded that patients with a history of 3 or more attacks of diverticulitis are at greatest risk for uncomplicated recurrence.

Several other earlier studies have been conducted to analyse the risk factors for overall and complicated recurrence of acute diverticulitis. These studies have suggested several factors associated with increased recurrence. These include C-reactive protein [9, 10] age over 50 years [9, 10], history of diverticulitis [9] family history of diverticulitis [11] male sex [12] corticosteroid use [13] and retroperitoneal abscess [8, 10]. Several studies have reported increased risk of complicated recurrence in patients using corticosteroid medication [12–15]; prophylactic sigmoid resection is probably warranted in these patients with lower threshold [16]. Patients with corticosteroid medication are also at higher risk for mortality due to complicated diverticulitis [17].

In conclusion, the risk score provides an easy and straightforward tool to predict complicated recurrence of diverticulitis. Uncomplicated recurrence is likely if a patient already has had three or more attacks of diverticulitis before.

RECURRENCE IN IMMUNOCOMPROMISED PATIENTS

Although rate of recurrence in immunocompromised patients is same as that of immunocompetent patients (20.5% vs 18.5%), but the severity of attacks is more in immunocompromised patients (87.5% vs 29.4%). This has been confirmed in several studies conducted by Samdani et al. and Biondo et al. [18, 19]. Patients who are immunocompromised have been reported to have a higher chance of emergency surgery during a recurrent episode (75% vs 23.5%) and also a higher need of an intestinal stoma during second surgery (100% vs 25%). Overall mortality during the recurrent episode has also been reported higher in patients who had received chemotherapy.

In a study conducted by Biondo et al. [19], a total of 931 patients were recruited between 1994 to 2008, out of which 166 were immunocompromised and 765 were immunocompetent. Recurrence rates were studied in these patients over a follow-up period of 81.62 months. A total of 136 patients (20.7%) developed one or more episodes of acute diverticulitis which included 21.5% of the immunocompromised patients and 20.5% of the immunocompetent ones. 16.4% patients had one recurrence, 3% had two and 1.3% had three or more recurrent episodes. There was no significant statistical difference between the two groups. Immunocompromised patients with a severe first episode did show a significant higher recurrence rate as well as more severe recurrent episodes. However, there were no differences with immunocompetent patients regarding need for emergency surgery. Recurrence rates were found highest during the first 6 months. These patients are very often offered a surgical treatment even after the first attack of diverticulitis. However they carry a poor prognosis after surgery due to immunocompromised state [20-23].

Risk of Recurrent Diverticulitis After Resection

There have been two studies which have shown similar results after the resection of sigmoid colon as far as the risk of diverticulitis is concerned [24-27]. In one such study, conducted at Mayo clinic by Benn and colleagues, 501 patients underwent sigmoid resection for diverticular disease. Out of 501 patient, anastomosis was performed at the distal sigmoid colon in 302 patients. Out of 302 patients, 12.55% patients had recurrent diverticulitis. In 180 patients, anastomosis was performed in proximal rectum. Out of which, recurrent diverticulitis was seen in 6.7% patients. In another study conducted at Cleveland clinic, 236 patients underwent sigmoid colon resection for diverticular disease and the results were similar. The risk of recurrent diverticulitis was four times higher in patients who had colo-sigmoid anastomosis rather than colorectal anastomosis. Thus the authors concluded that to decrease the risk of recurrent diverticulitis, the distal resection margin should be the proximal rectum. It has been suggested by Coloproctologists of Great Britain and Ireland that splenic flexure should be routinely mobilized as it helps in tension free anastomosis in already foreshortened colon due to diverticular disease.

Treatment of Recurrent Diverticulitis

Till recently it was believed that recurrent episodes of diverticulitis lead to complicated diverticulitis and higher mortality [28]. However, multiple studies have been conducted that have failed to prove the same. The overall mortality rate for patients with a previous history of diverticulitis has been reported as 2.5%, in contrast to a mortality rate of 10% seen in patients with a first attack of complicated diverticulitis [29]. It was also believed that elective sigmoid resection for diverticulitis is associated with high risk of mortality (2.3%) and high risk of colostomy (14.2%) [30-32]. Furthermore, the risk of recurrent diverticulitis is not eliminated after sigmoid resection and the recurrence rates may vary between 2.6% and 10.4% [32].

After considering above facts, in 2006, the American Society of Colon and Rectal Surgeons revised their recommendations and recommended an individualized approach to patients after an attack of acute diverticulitis [33]. Nowadays, conservative treatment has become the preferred choice after an episode of diverticulitis [33].

MEDICAL STRATEGIES IN PREVENTING DIVERTICULITIS RECURRENCE

Several high-quality randomized trials and systematic reviews have been carried out to provide strategy and guidelines to prevent recurrence of diverticulitis. Despite the lack of evidence from these high-quality studies, various dietary modifications and medications have been suggested to control the recurrence.

High-Fibre Diet

After an acute attack has resolved patient is usually advised to maintain high fibre diet to optimise the bowel movements [6]. However, the role of dietary modification in prevention of recurrent diverticulitis is unclear [34-36]. Consumption of seeds, popcorn and nuts should be avoided, based on the assumption that such substances could enter into the diverticulum and block or irritate it, resulting into diverticulitis, and possibly increasing the risk of perforation [28]. However no data is available at present to support this practice [37].

Non Absorbable Antibiotics

It has now been understood that there is an imbalance of microbiota in the pathogenesis of diverticulitis as a result of which the role of a non-absorbable antibiotic, Rifaximin has come to the surface. Thus in preventing the diverticulitis relapse and preventing its complications, cyclic treatment with Rifaximin has been proposed [38, 39].

Lanas et al. [40] recently conducted a multicentre, randomized, open controlled study in patients with a recent episode of colonic diverticulitis currently in remission and studied the role of the rifaximin in preventing recurrence of diverticulitis. Patients were divided into two groups. One group received 3.5 g of high-fibre supplementation twice a day with or without one week per month of rifaximin in dose of 400 mg twice a day for 12 months, while as another group received fibre alone. Recurrence of diverticulitis was seen in 10.4% of patients who received Rifaximin plus fibre as compared to 19.3% of patients who received fibre alone. The results were statistically significant in favour of using Rifaximin plus fibre.

5-Aminosalicylic-Acid

In case of an acute inflammation there is always a need to stop the inflammatory process in diverticulitis. 5-aminosalicylic acid (5-ASA) agents, which are anti-inflammatory agents have been used to prevent recurrent diverticulitis. Some randomized clinical trials (RCTs) have been conducted to investigate the role of 5-aminosalicylic acid (5-ASA). However, the efficacy results for secondary prevention in uncomplicated diverticulitis differed across studies. It has been found the mechanism responsible for inflammation in diverticulitis may be similar to that of inflammatory bowel disease [40]. This hypothesis has been proved on following observations and all patients with any of these proinflammatory situations are at higher risk of diverticulitis recurrence. These observations include:

- An increased concentration of inflammatory infiltrate along with enhanced expression of pro-inflammatory cytokines have been found in diverticular disease depending on the severity of the disease [41, 42].

- Obesity has been reported is an important risk factor for recurrent diverticulitis due to the pro inflammatory effect of the adipokynes and chemokynes [43, 44]
- Persistent abdominal pain is seen in up to 20% of patients after surgical treatment of diverticulitis which has an overall bad effect on quality of life of these patients [44]. These persistent symptoms are believed to be due to an increased level of neuropeptides found in mucosal biopsies of these patients and is an indicator of resolved prior acute inflammation and persistent chronic inflammation [45].

Mesalazine and its prodrug balsalazide, alone or in combination with an antibiotic or probiotics, have been found effective in preventing recurrence of diverticulitis [46, 47]. This is based on the hypothesis that Mesalazine reduces the inflammatory infiltrate and decreases the expression of proinflammatory cytokine [48]. Mesalazine has been found to be superior to rifaximin because mesalazine is believed to reduce endoscopic and histological inflammation after an attack of acute diverticulitis [49-52]. Mesalzine has been found to provide good relief from pain and other symptoms and have been found to be effective in preventing recurrence of diverticulitis [53-55].

Probiotics

Probiotics are living microorganisms that alter the host microflora and exert specific health benefits without increasing the risk of antibiotic resistance. These Probiotic microorganisms have multiple modes of action which include inhibiting the adherence of pathogens, improving mucosal defence, stimulating secretion of immunoglobulin A in Peyer's patches, decreasing bacterial translocation,, and enhancing immune system activity by controlling the balance of pro- and anti-inflammatory cytokines [56].

In the last few years, several studies have been conducted to evaluate the role of probiotics in the treatment of diverticular disease [57-60]. In one of such studies carried out 10 years before, Giaccari et al. [57] administered the combination of non-absorbable antibiotic, Rifaximin and Lactobacillus probiotic in 79 patients with post diverticulitis colonic stenosis. They found that 88% of the 79 patients remained symptom free for a period of 12-months. No repeated episodes of diverticulitis occurred during the follow-up period and stenosis improved or remained stable in 50% of patients.

Recently a study was carried out to investigate the role of combination of balsalazide, a 5-aminosalicylic acid prodrug, with a high-potency and a probiotic mixture VSL#3 in preventing recurrence of diverticulitis. VSL#3 probiotic is a mixture of eight different bacterial strains which include L. casei, L. plantarum, L. acidophilus, L. delbrueckii subsp. bulgaricus, B. longum, B. breve, B. infantis, Streptococcus salivarius and subsp. thermophiles) [47]. The authors found that the combination of balsalazide and VSL#3 was better than VSL#3 alone in preventing relapse of uncomplicated diverticulitis of the colon, although it had no statistical significance.

Surgical Management

Previously, the surgery in diverticulitis was recommended after two attacks of uncomplicated diverticulitis or after one attack of complicated diverticulitis, or after one attack in patients under the age of 40 years. Now the recommendations are individualized based on disease related factors, severity of recurrent attacks of diverticulitis, the risk of perforation and need for emergency surgery and risk of development of complicated diverticulitis. However the main reasons for surgical intervention in patients with recurrent diverticulitis are to prevent further attacks of diverticulitis, thereby improving the quality of life, to prevent the potential complications like colo-vesical fistula or colovaginal fistula and to prevent the potential risk of emergency colostomy formation.

Surgical Technique and Preoperative Assessment

Elective-Resection

The goal of management in case of acute diverticulitis should be to convert emergent or urgent operation into an elective procedure so as to minimize the chances of post-operative complications [61, 62]. After it has been decided that an elective sigmoid resection is to be done, a 4-6 weeks should be allowed to allow the inflammation to subside so as to increase the chances of complete single stage resection with lesser possible complications. Unfortunately emergency surgery cannot be postponed in some situations and in these cases the magnitude of intraperitoneal contamination indicates the choice of reconstruction. The Hinchey's classification is widely used to access the degree of contamination.

Though many people don't recommend preoperative bowel preparation but some do suggest bowel preparation prior to surgery. Proponents of bowel preparation believe that it makes the handling of colon easy and also facilitates the application of staplers. Recent studies show that preoperative administration of antibiotics decreases the chances of wound site infection. It is also recommended that patients with hydronephrosis secondary to inflammatory phlegmon should undergo prior stenting.

Generally, with localized contamination whether stage I or stage II, primary anastomosis without a protective colostomy can be performed. While with more diffuse contamination as in grade III and grade IV, a two-staged procedure is generally preferred. The two-staged procedures are either a Hartmann's procedure or a primary anastomosis with a protective proximal diverting stoma. Single stage sigmoid resection can either be done by open approach or laparoscopic approach. The latter minimises the post-operative hospital stay with quick recovery and less post-operative pain. Recent data suggests that laparoscopic surgery is associated with lesser operative site infections, lesser chances of ileus and lesser post-operative adhesion formation.

Open-Sigmoid Colectomy

For open sigmoid colectomy, patient is positioned in lithotomy position after inserting the Foleys catheter. Abdomen is opened via a vertical midline incision. Colon is rotated medially and lateral to medial approach is used by incising line of Toldt. In case of phlegmon the ureter and gonadal vessels are difficult to identify. It is wiser to stay close to bowel and not to resect more mesentery. It has been shown in some studies that taking care of superior rectal artery will prevent anastomotic leak by improving blood flow thereby decreasing the risk of anastomotic leak.

Laparoscopic Sigmoid Colectomy

In case of laparoscopic procedures, preoperative considerations are similar to open surgery. Patient is placed in split leg table with legs abducted or in modified lithotomy position. The patient is secured with the table with arms tucked. Port placement depends on surgeon's preference and anatomy of the patient, but generally includes a supra-umbilical port, right and left lower quadrant ports and right upper quadrant port. Mobilization of colon depends on surgeon's preference and could be medial to lateral or lateral to medial.

For lateral to medial approach, recto-sigmoid and sigmoid colon is retracted medially and incision is made along the line of toldt and continued up to the splenic flexure and down towards the sacral promontory or recto sigmoid junction. The ureter and gonadal vessels are identified. Peritoneum is incised and window created to ligate the inferior mesenteric vessels. The ureter can be confused with superior rectal artery and both should be identified prior to transaction.

There has been a trend for mobilization from medial to lateral side in laparoscopic surgery which helps in creating a space between retro peritoneum and mesocolon. Inferior mesenteric artery is identified and ligated. The surgeon should be familiar with both the techniques though both the techniques are equally good. In case of recurrent diverticulitis because of inflammatory phlegmon formation and shortened mesentery, laparoscopic technique may be difficult at times and it may be difficult to complete the procedure and conversion to open is demanded. Air leak test should be preferably done as routine in all the cases after completion of procedure.

Hand Assisted Laparoscopic Sigmoid Colectomy

Hand assisted laparoscopic sigmoid resection takes lesser time then complete laparoscopic procedure without any compromise on final outcome [63, 64]. In cases of fibrosis or phlegmon, insertion of hand makes the procedure easy to accomplish as hand can be used to break the adhesions and for blunt dissection and mobilization of colon. A lower conversion rate has been shown by many studies in hand assisted laparoscopic procedures as compared to purely laparoscopic procedures. In the situations where conversion to open is demanded, hand assisted procedure may be a better alternative to avert the conversion.

Emergency Procedures

Hartman's Procedure

Though Hartman's procedure was initially devised for carcinoma rectum in 1923 as an alternative to abdomino-perineal resection, it is now considered as procedure of choice for most of the cases of perforated diverticulosis who need emergency surgery. This procedure has replaced the three stage procedure of initial colostomy, with subsequent resection and colostomy takedown. This procedure is being routinely performed for patients with perforated diverticulitis associated with purulent peritonitis or faecal peritonitis [65, 66].

References

[1] Boles, RS, Jr. and Jordan, SM. (1958). The clinical significance of diverticulosis. *Gastroenterology*, 35:579–582. [PubMed] [Google Scholar].

[2] Zollinger, RW. (1968). The prognosis in diverticulitis of the colon. *Arch Surg,* 97: 418–422. [PubMed] [Google Scholar].

[3] Rodkey GV. and Welch CE. (1984). Changing patterns in the surgical treatment of diverticular disease. *Ann Surg*, 200:466–478. [PMC free article] [PubMed] [Google Scholar].

[4] Hupfeld, L., Pommergaard, HC, Burcharth, J. and Rosenberg, J. (July, 2018). Emergency admissions for complicated colonic diverticulitis are increasing: a nationwide register-based cohort study. *Int J Colorectal Dis*, 33(7):879–86.

[5] El-Sayed, C., Radley, S., Mytton, J., Evison, F. and Ward ST. (March, 2018). Risk of Recurrent Disease and Surgery Following an Admission for Acute Diverticulitis. *Dis Colon Rectum*, 61(3):382–9.

[6] Sallinen, V., Mali, J., Cand, M., Leppäniemi, A. and Mentula, P. (Feb. 2015). Assessment of Risk for Recurrent Diverticulitis; A Proposal of Risk Score for Complicated Recurrence. *Medicine (Baltimore)*, 94(8): e557. Published online 2015 Feb 27. doi: 10.1097/MD. 0000000000000557, PMCID: PMC4554145.

[7] Chapman, JR., Dozois, EJ. and Wolff, BG. (2006). Diverticulitis: a progressive disease? Do multiple recurrences predict less favourable outcomes? *Ann Surg,* 243:876–883. [PMC free article] [PubMed] [Google Scholar].

[8] Hall, JF., Roberts, PL. and Ricciardi R. (2011). Long-term follow-up after an initial episode of diverticulitis: what are the predictors of recurrence? *Dis Colon Rectum,* 54:283–288. [PubMed] [Google Scholar].

[9] Anaya, DA. and Flum, DR. (2005). Risk of emergency colectomy and colostomy in patients with diverticular disease. *Arch Surg*, 140:681–685. [PubMed] [Google Scholar].

[10] Buchs, NC., Konrad-Mugnier. B. and Jannot AS. (2013). Assessment of recurrence and complications following uncomplicated diverticulitis. *Br J Surg*, 100:976–979. [PubMed] [Google Scholar].

[11] Kim, SY., Oh, TH. and Seo JY. (2012). The clinical factors for predicting severe diverticulitis in Korea: a comparison with Western

countries. *Gut Liver,* 6:78. [PMC free article] [PubMed] [Google Scholar].

[12] Hjern, F., Mahmood, MW. and Abraham-Nordling, M. (2015). Cohort study of Corticosteroid use and risk of hospital admission for diverticular disease. *Br J Surg*, 102:119– 124. [PubMed] [Google Scholar].

[13] Klarenbeek, BR., Samuels, M. and van der Wal, MA. (2010). Indications for elective sigmoid resection in diverticular disease. *Ann Surg,* 251:670–674. [PubMed] [Google Scholar].

[14] Yoo, PS., Garg, R, and Salamone, LF. (2008). Medical comorbidities predict the need for Colectomy for complicated and recurrent diverticulitis. *Am J Surg*, 196:710–714. [PubMed] [Google Scholar].

[15] Curtis, JR., Xie, F. and Chen L. (2011). The incidence of gastrointestinal perforations among rheumatoid arthritis patients. *Arthritis Rheum,* 63:346–351. [PMC free article] [PubMed] [Google Scholar].

[16] Morris, AM., Regenbogen, SE. and Hardiman, KM. (2014). Sigmoid diverticulitis. *JAMA* 311:287. [PubMed] [Google Scholar].

[17] Chapman, J., Davies, M. and Wolff B. (2005) complicated diverticulitis: is it time to rethink the rules? *Ann Surg*, 242:576–581. [PMC free article] [PubMed] [Google Scholar].

[18] Samdani, T., Pieracci, FM., Eachempati, SR., Benarroch-Gampel, J., Weiss, A., Pietanza, MC., Barie, PS., and Nash, GM. (Dec. 2014). Colonic diverticulitis in chemotherapy patients: should operative indications change? A retrospective cohort study. *Int J Surg,* 12(12):1489-94. doi: 10.1016/j.ijsu.2014.10.032.

[19] Biondo, S., Borao, JL. and Kreisler E, et al. Recurrence and virulence of colonic diverticulitis in immunocompromised patients. *Am J Surg*. 2012;204: 172–9.

[20] Scotti, M., Santangelo, S., Federico, R., Carrano, C., La Tessa, N., Carlomagno, DG., Palmieri, A.. Calogero, M., Piantadosi, and A, Renda. (Sep. 2014). Complicated diverticulitis in kidney transplanted patients: Analysis of 717 cases. *Transplant Proc*. 46(7): 2247- 2250. doi: 10.1016/j.transproceed.2014.07.044.

[21] Perkins, JD., Shield, CF III., Chang, FC. and Farha, GJ. (1984). Acute diverticulitis: comparison of treatment in immune-compromised and non-immunocompromised patients. *Am J Surg,* 148:745–748.

[22] Al-Khamis, A., Abou, KJ., Demian M., Morin N., Carol-Ann,VH., Philip, G. and Boutros M. (Feb. 2016). Sigmoid Colectomy for Acute Diverticulitis in Immunosuppressed vs Immunocompetent Patients: Outcomes from the ACS-NSQIP Database. *Dis Colon Rectum*, 59(2):101– 109, doi: 10.1097/DCR.0000000000000513.

[23] Al Harakeha, H., Pailyb, A J., Doughana, S. and Shaikhb I. (2018). Recurrent Acute Diverticulitis: When to Operate? *Inflamm. Intest. Dis*, 3:91–99. www.karger.com/i,id doi: 10.1159/00049497.

[24] Raskin, JB. (2012). *Prevention of Recurrence of Diverticulitis* (PREVENT 2) (NCT00545103). Available at: http://www.clinicaltrials.gov/ct2/show/{"type":"clinical-trial", "attrs":{"text":"NCT00545103","term_id":"NCT00545103"}}NCT00545103.

[25] Richards, R. and Hammitt, J. (2002). Timing of prophylactic surgery in prevention of diverticulitis recurrence: a cost-effectiveness analysis. *Dig Dis Sci*, 47: 1903–1908 [PubMed] [Google Scholar].

[26] Salem, L., Veenstra, D., Sullivan, S. and Flum, D. (2004). The timing of elective colectomy in diverticulitis: a decision analysis. *J Am Coll Surg,* 199: 904–912 [PubMed] [Google Scholar].

[27] Scarpa, M., Pagano, D., Ruffolo, C., Pozza, A., Polese, L. and Frego,M. (2009) Health-related quality of life after colonic resection for diverticular disease: long-term results. *J Gastrointest Surg*, 13: 105–112 [PubMed] [Google Scholar].

[28] Stollman, N. and Raskin J. (1999). Diagnosis and management of diverticular disease of the colon in adults: Ad Hoc Practice Parameters Committee of the American College of Gastroenterology. *Am J Gastro enterol*, 94: 3110–3121.

[29] Chautems, R., Ambrosetti, P., Ludwig, A., Mermillod, B., Morel, P. and Soravia C. (2002). Long term follow-up after first acute episode of sigmoid diverticulitis: is surgery mandatory? A prospective study of 118 patients. *Dis Colon Rectum,* 45: 962–966 [PubMed] [Google Scholar].

[30] Hart, A., Kennedy, H., Stebbings, W. and Day N. (2002). How frequently do large bowel diverticula perforate? An incidence and cross-sectional study. *Eur J Gastroenterol Hepatol,* 12: 661–666 [PubMed] [Google Scholar].

[31] Richards, R. and Hammitt J. (2002). Timing of prophylactic surgery in prevention of diverticulitis recurrence: a cost-effectiveness analysis. *Dig Dis Sci,* 47: 1903–1908 [PubMed] [Google Scholar].

[32] Salem, L., Veenstra, D., Sullivan, S. and Flum D. (2004). The timing of elective colectomy in diverticulitis: a decision analysis. *J Am Coll Surg*, 199: 904–912 [PubMed] [Google Scholar].

[33] Rafferty, J., Shellito, P., Hyman, N. and Buie, W. (2006). Standards Committee of American Society of Colon and Rectal Surgeons; Practice parameters for sigmoid diverticulitis. *Dis Colon Rectum,* 49: 939–944 [PubMed] [Google Scholar.

[34] Crowe, F., Appleby, P., Allen, N. and Key, T. (2011). Diet and risk of diverticular disease in Oxford cohort of European Prospective Investigation into Cancer and Nutrition (EPIC): Prospective study of British vegetarians and non-vegetarians. *BMJ* 343: d4131. [PMC free article] [PubMed] [Google Scholar].

[35] Murphy, T., Hunt, R., Fried, M. and Krabshuis, J. (2007). World Gastroenterology Organisation practice guidelines: diverticular disease. Milwaukee: *WGO*;1-16. [Google Scholar].

[36] Peery, A., Barrett, P., Park, D., Rogers, A., Galanko, J., Martin C. et al. (2012). A high-fiber diet does not protect against asymptomatic diverticulosis. *Gastroenterology*, 142: 266– 272 [PMC free article] [PubMed] [Google Scholar].

[37] Strate, L., Liu, Y., Syngal, S., Aldoori, W. and Giovannucci, E. (2008). Nut, corn, and popcorn consumption and the incidence of diverticular disease. *JAMA*, 300: 907–914 [PMC free article] [PubMed] [Google Scholar].

[38] Tursi, A., Elisei, W., Brandimarte, G., Giorgetti, G. and Aiello, F. (2010) Predictive value of serologic markers of degree of histologic damage in acute uncomplicated colonic diverticulitis. *J Clin Gastroenterol*, 44: 702–706.

[39] Bianchi, M., Festa, V., Moretti, A., Ciaco, A., Mangone, M., Tornatore V. et al. (2011). Meta-analysis: long-term therapy with rifaximin in the management of uncomplicated diverticular disease. *Aliment Pharmacol Ther*, 33: 902–910.

[40] Lanas, A., Ponce, J., Bignamini, A. and Mearin F. (2013). One year intermittent rifaximin plus fibre supplementation vs. fibre supplementation alone to prevent diverticulitis recurrence: a proof-of-concept study. *Dig Liver Dis* 45: 104–109 [PubMed] [Google Scholar].

[41] Tursi, A., Brandimarte, G., Elisei, W., Giorgetti, G., Inchingolo, C., Danese, S., et al. (2008a). Assessment and grading of mucosal inflammation in colonic diverticular disease. *J. Clin Gastroenterol,* 42: 699–703.

[42] Tursi, A., Elisei, W., Brandimarte, G., Giorgetti,G., Inchingolo, C. and Nenna, R., et al. (May, 2012). Musosal tumour necrosis factor-alpha in diverticular disease of the colon is over expressed with disease severity. *Colorectal Dis,* 14(5):e258-63. doi: 10.1111/j.1463-1318. 2012.02926.x.

[43] Batra, A. and Siegmund B. (2012). The role of visceral fat. *Dig Dis,* 30: 70–74.

[44] Tursi, A., Elisei, W., Giorgetti, G., Inchingolo, C., Nenna, R. and Picchio M., et al. (2013) Effectiveness of different therapeutic strategies in preventing diverticulitis recurrence. *Eur Rev Med Pharmacol Sci,* 17: 342–34.

[45] Bargellini, T., Martellucci, J., Tonelli, P., Valeri, A. (2013). Long-term results of treatment of acute diverticulitis: still lessons to be learned? *Updates Surg,* 65: 125–130.

[46] Tursi, A., Brandimarte, G. and Daffinaà, R. (2002). Long-term treatment with mesalazine and rifaximin versus rifaximin alone for patients with recurrent attacks of acute diverticulitis of colon. *Dig Liver Dis*, 34: 510–515 [PubMed] [Google Scholar].

[47] Tursi, A., Brandimarte, G., Giorgetti, G., Elisei, W. and Aiello F. (2007). Balsalazide and/or high-potency probiotic mixture (VSL#3) in maintaining remission after attack of acute, uncomplicated

diverticulitis of the colon. *Int. J. Colorectal Dis* 22: 1103–1108 [PubMed] [Google Scholar].

[48] Tursi, A., Elisei, W., Brandimarte, G., Giorgetti, G., Inchingolo, C., Nenna R., et al. (2012). Mucosal expression of basic fibroblastic growth factor, Syndecan 1 and tumor necrosis factor-alpha in diverticular disease of the colon: a case-control study. *Neuro gastroenterol Motil*, 24: 836–e396 [PubMed] [Google Scholar.

[49] Tursi, A., Elisei, E., Giorgetti, G., Inchingolo, C., Nenna, R. Picchio M., et al. (2013) Detection of endoscopic and histological inflammation after an attack of colonic diverticulitis is associated with higher diverticulitis recurrence. *J Gastrointest Liver Dis,* 22: 12–17, [PubMed] [Google Scholar].

[50] Tursi, A., Elisei, W., Giorgetti, G., Inchingolo, C., Nenna, R.,Picchio M., et al. (2013) Effectiveness of different therapeutic strategies in preventing diverticulitis recurrence. *Eur Rev Med Pharmacol Sci,* 17: 342–348 [PubMed] [Google Scholar].

[51] Lombardo, L. and Lapertosa G. (1991). The ambulatory medical treatment of colonic diverticulitis. An open clinico-endoscopic-histological study with rifaximin, a non-aminoglycoside enteric antibiotic. *Recenti Prog Med.* 82: 300–304 [PubMed] [Google Scholar].

[52] Tursi, A., and Papagrigoriadis, S. (2009). Review article: The current and evolving treatment of colonic diverticular disease. *Aliment Pharmacol Ther.* 30: 532–546 [PubMed] [Google Scholar].

[53] Smith, J., Humes, D., Garsed, K., Lam, C., Zaitoun, A. and Bennett A., et al. (2012). Mechanistic randomised control trial of mesalazine in symptomatic diverticular disease. *Gut,* 61: A51–A52 [Google Scholar].

[54] Gaman, A., Teodorescu,R., Georghescu, E. and Abagiu M. (2011). Diverticular disease: a fresh approach to a neglected disease. In: *Folk Symposium 178, Cologne, Germany,* 2–3 [Google Scholar].

[55] Kruis, W., Meier, E., Schumacher, M., Mickisch, O., Greinwald, R. and Mueller R. (2013). The German SAG-20 Study Group; Randomised clinical trial: mesalazine (Salofalk granules) for

uncomplicated diverticular disease of the colon – a placebo-controlled study. *Aliment Pharmacol Ther,* 37: 680–690 [Pu56). bMed] [Google Scholar].

[56] Gionchetti, P., Amadini, C., Rizzello, F., Venturi, A., Palmonari, V., Morselli, C. et al. (2002). Probiotics – role in inflammatory bowel disease. *Dig Liver Dis*. 34(Suppl. 2): S58–S62, [PubMed] [Google Scholar].

[57] Giaccari, S., Tronci, S., Falconieri, M. and Ferrieri, A. (1993). Long-term treatment with Rifaximin and lactobacilli in post-diverticulitic stenosis of the colon. *Eur Rev Med Pharmacol Sci.* 15: 29–34 [PubMed] [Google Scholar].

[58] Unlu, Ç., Daniels, L., Vrouenraets, B. and Boermeester, M. (2012). Systematic review of medical therapy to prevent recurrent diverticulitis. *Int J Colorectal Dis* 27: 1131–1136 [PubMed] [Google Scholar].

[59] Zullo, A., Hassan, C., Maconi, G., Manes, G., Tammaro, G., De Francesco, V. et al. (2010). Cyclic antibiotic therapy for diverticular disease: a critical reappraisal. *J Gastrointestin Liver Dis,* 19: 295–302 [PubMed] [Google Scholar].

[60] Weizman A. and Nguyen G. (2011). Diverticular disease: epidemiology and management. *Can J Gastroenterol,* 25: 385–389 [PMC free article] [PubMed] [Google Scholar].

[61] Oberkofler, CE., Rickenbacher, A. and Raptis DA. (2012). A multicenter randomized clinical trial of primary anastomosis or Hartmann's procedure for perforated left colonic diverticulitis with purulent or fecal peritonitis. *Ann Surg,* 256(5):819-826; discussion 826-817.

[62] Bridoux, V., Regimbeau, JM. and Ouaissi, M. (2017). Hartmann's Procedure or Primary Anastomosis for Generalized Peritonitis due to Perforated Diverticulitis: A Prospective Multicenter Randomized Trial (DIVERTI). *J Am Coll Surg.* 225(6):798-805.

[63] Benn, PL., Wolff,BG. and Ilstrup, DM. (1986). Level of anastomosis and recurrent colonic diverticulitis. *Am J Surg,*151(2):269-271.

[64] Cirocchi, R., Afshar, S. and Di Saverio, S. (2017). A historical review of surgery for peritonitis secondary to acute colonic diverticulitis: from Lockhart-Mummery to evidence-based medicine. *World J Emerg Surg*. 2017;12:14.

[65] Stumpf, MJ., Vinces, FY. and Edwards. J. (2007). Is primary anastomosis safe in the surgical management of complications of acute diverticulitis? *Am Surg,* 73(8):787-790; discussion 790-781.

[66] Balanzoni, S., Perrucci, A., Pasi, L. and Montanari, MC. (1997). The Hartmann intervention. The current indications and the authors' own experience]. *Minerva Chir,*52(4):383-386.

In: Diverticulitis: Diagnosis and Treatment
ISBN: 978-1-53618-081-7
Editors: Shams-ul-Bari et al.

Chapter 9

DIVERTICULITIS: RECENT ADVANCES

Fazl Q. Parray* and Gowher Aziz Bhat
Sher-I-Kashmir Institute of Medical Sciences,
Soura, Srinagar, J&K, India

ABSTRACT

Management strategies for diverticulitis are under constant debate, appraisal and evolution. Colonoscopy in uncomplicated acute diverticulitis is controversial but mandatory after complicated episodes. Diverticulitis is challenging that demands clinicians to provide an individualized yet evidence-based approach. Newer technologies for diagnosis and new guidelines for management have emerged and resulted in better outcome. Newer concepts of pathogenesis, implicating inflammation, microbiome shifts, visceral hypersensitivity, and abnormal motility are influencing the management strategies in a significant way.

* Corresponding Author's Email: fazlparray@rediffmail.com, fazlparray@gmail.com.

INTRODUCTION

Acute diverticulitis is an important cause of frequent outpatient visits and hospital admissions. This disease entity is a significant brunt on health care costs and statistically accounts for approximately 200000 hospital admissions every year. Annual costs of diverticular disease are estimated at $2.7 billion per year in the United States [1, 2]. Around 4% patients with diverticulosis develop diverticulitis. Approximately >75% of the patients with diverticulitis report with uncomplicated disease, whereas rest of the 20-25% with complicated disease. Many patients present to medical centres time and again with a variety of symptoms. These patients present with significant morbidity and impact on quality of life (QOL). About 80% patients with complicated diverticulitis respond to conservative management, while as rest of the 20% patients need surgery.

New concepts of pathogenesis, implicating inflammation, microbiome shifts, visceral hypersensitivity, and abnormal motility are influencing the management strategies [3, 4]. In this chapter we will be briefly discussing the various controversies and recent advances for the management of diverticulitis.

DIAGNOSTIC MODALITIES

Imaging

CT scan is the gold standard of imaging. The accuracy is further enhanced if oral, intravenous and rectal contrast is used. This imaging modality is highly sensitive and specific with low false positive rate. In CT images one can identify diverticulae as extraluminal air or fluid, colonic wall thickening >4 mm and abscess formation. CT images at the same time help in diagnosing any associated findings like liver abscess, pyelo-phelibitis, strictures, obstruction and colovesical fistula. In mild diverticulitis CT images shows localized wall thickening (>5 mm) and inflammation of pericolic fat. In severe diverticulitis CT images show localized wall thickening, with inflammation of pericolic fat, with abscess and extra luminal air or contrast [5].

CT FINDINGS CLASSIFIED ON BASIS OF MODIFIED HINCHEY CLASSIFICATION SYSTEM

- Stage 0 - Mild clinical diverticulitis
- Stage 1a - Confined pericolic inflammation, phlegmon
- Stage 1b- Confined pericolic abscess (within sigmoid mesocolon)
- Stage 2 - Pelvic, distant intra-abdominal or intra-peritoneal abscess
- Stage 3 - Generalised purulent peritonitis
- Stage 4 - Faecal peritonitis

Severity of disease on CT may allow the selection of patients who will most likely respond to conservative therapy. Sigmoid resection is recommended for selected patients only, particularly with more complex and large abscess or those with fistula.

Colonoscopy

There is still a controversy for timing of colonoscopy after an acute attack. Ideally it should be avoided in acute diverticulitis because of the risk of perforation. Colonoscopy should be performed 6 to 8 weeks after inflammation subsides. It confirms the diagnosis and excludes malignancy.

Imaging Sensitivity

CT scan can aid in distinguishing carcinoma from diverticulitis after an acute attack. CT colonography should be considered in such cases which has a sensitivity of 98% when compared to barium enema (BE) with a sensitivity of 92%. Strictures in diverticulitis are usually longer and more regular than cancer.

DCR reports a study by Australian Group on 1088 patients with diverticulitis. A total of 319 patients underwent colonoscopy; out of which 23 (2.1%) were found to have cancer. Negative Predictive value of diverticulitis diagnosis by CT for colorectal cancer (CRC) is 97.9%; Odds of diagnosis of CRC were 6.7 times in patients with abscess, 4 times in patients with localised perforation and 18 times in patients with fistula. When the cohort was compared to their general population, the finding demonstrated that even though the overall risk is low but still had higher risk than general population, especially in younger patients and in complicated disease. Thus, the conclusion drawn from the study recommended routine colonoscopy in all cases of complicated diverticulitis [6].

Estimated Risk of Malignancy

Studies have shown that malignancy risk in uncomplicated disease is 0.7%, whereas the risk goes as high as 10.8% in complicated disease. The conclusion drawn was that risk of malignancy after radiographically proven episode of acute uncomplicated diverticulitis is low.

Recent Advances in Medical Management

Most patients with diverticulosis remain asymptomatic and usually do not need any kind of treatment. Some percentage of patients do develop diverticulitis, which may remain uncomplicated or get complicated at times. Because of these varied modes of presentation, a physician, radiologist, medical gastroenterologist, general surgeon or a colorectal surgeon may be involved in diagnostic evaluation and management of these patients. The management of patients with diverticulitis depends on their severity of presentation, presence of complications and comorbid conditions.

Uncomplicated diverticulitis can be managed medically in an ambulatory setting. Complicated disease requires a more aggressive approach. It can often require urgent or elective surgery and specific treatments like abscess drainage for complications [7].

ANTIBIOTICS

Patients with Hinchey stage 0 and Ia disease, are considered uncomplicated and can be treated on outpatient basis with clear liquid diet for 2-3 days, low fiber diet as tolerated, oral broad spectrum like ciprofloxacin plus metronidazole, moxifloxacin or amoxicillin clavulanate on a case to case basis along with acetaminophen and antispasmodics for pain control [7, 8].

In recent times the judicious use of antibiotics has been challenged after revisiting the pathophysiology which supports more of an inflammatory nature rather than infectious nature of diverticulitis [9, 10]. Even though the Cochrane review 2014 was not in favour of omitting the antibiotics but the guidelines at that time remained same [11].

However, some of the recent studies are in favour of not prescribing any antibiotics. The AVOD trial, which was a multicentre randomized controlled trial conducted in 10 surgical departments in Sweden &Iceland on 623 patients with CT proved diverticulitis, compared antibiotic arm versus no antibiotic arm. Complication rates remained same (1.9% vs. 1.0%) and length of stay also remained same (3 days). The conclusion drawn was that antibiotics for acute uncomplicated diverticulitis neither accelerate recovery nor prevent complications or recurrence. Antibiotics should be reserved for the treatment of complicated diverticulitis [12].

Amongst the patients allocated to non-antibiotic arm, 32% needed antibiotics because of increasing CRP level, fever and abdominal pain. Similarly in antibiotic arm or close Observation trial, 528 patients with a first episode of CT confirming left-sided uncomplicated acute diverticulitis (including those with Hinchey stages 1a–b [abscess size up to 5 cm] were randomized to antibiotic and no antibiotic arms. Patients in the antibiotic arm received a 10-day course of antibiotics. Supportive care in the no-antibiotic arm was not documented. The primary outcome, time to recovery, was defined as discharge from hospital, normal diet, temperature less than 38°C, visual analogue pain score below 4 (with no use of daily pain medication) and resumption of pre-illness working activities. This was similar between the 2 groups, as were secondary endpoints at long -term follow-up [13].

This evidence is incorporated in the "2017 American Gastroenterological Association (AGA) Institute Guideline on the Management of Acute Diverticulitis" which promotes selective individualised approach as opposed to routine use of antibiotics in this presentation [14].

MESALAZINE AND PROBIOTICS

The role of inflammation in the pathogenesis of diverticular disease is gaining popularity. The role of anti-inflammatory drugs like aminosalicyclate (5 ASA) and mesalazine has been investigated. However multiple placebo controlled trials have not been able to substantiate these facts [15, 16]. The findings were substantiated and reaffirmed by the results of eight randomized controlled trials in a 2017 systematic review and meta-analysis. 5 ASA compounds were not superior to controls for preventing recurrent attacks (RR 0.86, 95% CI 0.63–1.17) [17]. Alterations in the microbiome of the colon and dysbiosis have also been implicated in recurrent attacks and then targeted as a treatment focus with probiotics [18].

Rifaxamin, a poorly absorbed antibiotic, has been trialled both alone and in combination with fibre and/or mesalazine to modify this process. In a meta-analysis of 4 trials with 1,660 patients with symptomatic uncomplicated diverticular disease, treatment with rifaximin plus fibre supplementation was effective in obtaining symptom relief and preventing complications at 1 year [19].

The benefits of probiotics have been investigated. However, a systematic review of 11 studies by Lahner et al. found that the included studies were of insufficient level of evidence to draw meaningful conclusions [20].

Outpatient versus Inpatient Management

Patients of uncomplicated diverticulitis have been managed by treating physicians both on inpatient and outpatient basis. To know in real sense what is better for these patients, a multicentre randomized trial named as *DIVER Trial* which included 132 Patients from 5 Hospitals in Spain was carried to study outpatient versus hospital treatment of uncomplicated diverticulitis (CT Confirmed) with antibiotics. In both arms there was same rate of treatment failure. Overall health care cost per episode was 3 times lower in outpatient group with no difference in QOL. The trial concluded that outpatient treatment is safe and effective in selected patients with uncomplicated acute diverticulitis. This also helps in saving the cost of treatment without any negative influence on QOL [21].

A recent systematic review of 10 studies concluded that failure rates for primary treatment and recurrence rates are similar when treated on an inpatient or outpatient basis [22]. The included studies mention ambulatory care as an in-patient hospital stay up to 24 h only, with discharge in an out-patient setting either on oral or iv antibiotics. This is confirmed by a recent paper by Joliat et al. who employed a similar outpatient treatment strategy. These authors found that factors including increasing time to admission with CT, Ambrosetti score of 4 and free air around the colon were predictive of treatment failure [23].

Indications for hospital admission include, evidence of severe diverticulitis (i.e., systemic signs of infection or peritonitis), inability to tolerate oral hydration, failure of outpatient therapy (i.e., persistent or increasing fever, pain, or leucocytosis after 2-3 days), immunocompromised patients or patients with significant comorbidities and pain severe enough to require parenteral narcotic analgesia [24].

Modified Hinchey stage Ib II, III and IV are categorized as patients with complicated diverticular disease. Patients in Modified Hinchey stage Ib may require hospitalization along with a clear liquid diet, followed by low fibre and intravenous or oral antibiotics. This may be followed by elective surgical resection or percutaneous drainage of abscess >4 cm, although abscess <3 cm will resolve with antibiotics alone. Modified Hinchey stages

II-IV require hospitalization. They should be prescribed nothing by mouth, intravenous antibiotics, and percutaneous abscess drainage. While as elective procedures are to be planned for patients in stage II, emergent or urgent surgical resection is needed for those in stage III and IV.

Monotherapy with carbapenems like piperacillin/tazobactam, ticarcillin/clavulanic acid, or ertapenem is appropriate for moderately ill patients [25] while as monotherapy with meropenem, imipenem-cilastatin, piperacillin-tazobactam, or doripenem should be prescribed in severely ill patients or who are immune-compromised.

Controversies in Surgical Treatment

Most perforations and complications do not occur after recurrences but at first attack. Thus an elective resection after recovery from uncomplicated disease may not decrease likelihood of later emergent surgery. After first attack, approximately 1/3rd patients will have second attack, while as after second attack further 1/3rd will have yet another attack. Conservative management of recurrent non-perforated diverticulitis is associated with better recovery and low morbidity and mortality. Thus the guidelines were revised in 2006 to a more conservative approach [26, 27].

Elective Sigmoid Resection

The decision to recommend elective sigmoid colectomy after recovery from acute diverticulitis should be made on a case to case basis. It is influenced by age, medical condition/comorbidities, frequency and severity of attacks. Patients with complicated disease, several recurrences and strong preferences will still need an elective resection in most cases, although surgery can usually be delayed by initial antibiotics and percutaneous abscess drainage. Laparoscopic lavage may buy some time in cases of purulent peritonitis and may help in converting an emergent operation into an elective or semi-elective surgery but patients with faecal peritonitis will still require an emergent operation. Even in the acute setting, if resection is indicated, one can consider a primary anastomosis with temporary loop ileostomy. Further research may better delineate which patients may still benefit from a more conservative approach [28].

In diverticulitis one usually comes across a thickened grossly diseased, adherent or a woody bowel, at times adherent to left ureter. Dissection should be careful and meticulous to release sigmoid colon. Proximal margin should be in complaint bowel and it is not important to include all the diverticulae proximally, however the distal margin should be through upper rectum to exclude the chances of recurrent disease in the residual sigmoid colon. Even a ureteral stenting preoperatively may be worthwhile in some cases to prevent ureteric injuries.

ELECTIVE SIGMOID RESECTION: IS BOWEL PREPARATION NECESSARY?

Bowel preparation has no influence on anastomotic leak rates or other septic complications as per the observation made by Netherlands group in a subgroup analysis of a multicentre (13 hospitals) randomized controlled trial; Out of 190 patients, undergoing sigmoid resections for diverticulitis, leak occurred in 7.8% prepared patients and in 5.7% unprepared patients. The conclusion of the study was that there was no significant difference in the groups with regard to anastomotic leak, septic complications and mortality [29].

Indications for Elective Sigmoid Resection

Mortality in patients of perforated diverticulitis is approximately 10%. A study was conducted to detect the risk factors associated with perforation in patients of diverticulitis. Patients with immunosuppression, chronic renal failure or cardiovascular disease were found to have 48% recurrence after successful conservative management.

The conclusion drawn was that elective sigmoid resection should be restricted and only considered in complicated cases and for high risk patients with immuno-suppression, chronic renal failure or cardiovascular disease, following a conservatively treated episode [30].

PREDICTING RECURRENCE AFTER INITIAL ATTACK

A retrospective study from Lahey group in 2011 concluded that recurrence of diverticulitis is common following an initial attack that has been managed medically and the complicated recurrence is uncommon. Patients with a family history of diverticulitis, long segment of involved colon, and/or retroperitoneal abscess are at higher risk for recurrent disease. Patients who present with right-sided diverticulitis are at low risk for recurrent disease. These findings should be taken into consideration when counselling patients regarding the potential benefits of prophylactic colectomy. Approximately 1/3rd of the patients will have a recurrence [31].

Operative Strategy

Three Stage Approach

The operative strategy for perforation with peritonitis (Hinchey III and IV) has changed. Initially a 3-stage operation was performed which includes diversion and drainage of the perforated area in stage one followed by resection of the affected area in stage two and finally reversal of stoma. 10-years' experience with this approach cited a mortality rate of 11% (78% of these deaths were related to the first procedure) [32].

Two Stage Approach

Hartman's procedure is performed in which the diseased segment is removed during the initial laparotomy [33] followed by reversal of Hartman in second stage. This became, and possibly still remains the standard of care, but the mortality has been cited as high as 15% [34]. Limitations of this procedure include mortality & morbidity of colostomy and life style implications of a permanent stoma [35].

One Stage Approach

Resection with restoration of continuity avoids some of these challenges. This surgery generates a concern about performing an anastomosis in a contaminated environment for a critically unwell patient. This would require a very selective approach. The overall mortality has been reported as 9.9 and 18.8% for primary anastomosis and Hartman's, respectively. Overall anastomotic leak rate for a primary anastomosis has been reported as 13.9%. Meta-analysis and direct comparisons could not be drawn due to heterogeneity [36].

This clinical question will be clarified further when the DIVA arm of the LADIES trial, a RCT comparing these 2 treatment modalities reports will be available.

Elective Surgery

There are at least two distinct indications for elective surgery. One is as a prophylaxis against recurrent attacks and complications and the second is surgery for ongoing symptoms that impact QOL. An initial enthusiasm for liberal pre-emptive elective surgery has somehow waned.

ASCRS guidelines recommended an elective resection after 1 or 2 episodes of acute uncomplicated diverticulitis in early days (Guidelines 2000) [37]. At present American Gastroenterology Association (AGA) advise against routine resection and instead propose an individualized approach [38]. Complications of diverticulitis typically manifest on the initial presentation. Morbidity and mortality of elective procedures for diverticulitis can be significant [39].

Laparoscopic Surgery

Patients report higher QOL scores and reduced abdominal symptoms after laparoscopic resections, but lacked direct comparisons with conservative management [40].

Ladies Trial

This is a MCRT (34 hospitals in Belgium, Netherlands, and Italy) aimed at investigating the acute surgical management of diverticulitis. The trial had 2 arms: DIVA arm and LOLA arm. DIVA arm compares resection plus end colostomy (Hartman's Procedure) to resection plus primary anastomosis. LOLA arm of this trial compared laparoscopic lavage to Hartman's procedure. In this study, 90 patients with purulent perforated diverticulitis were randomized to undergo either laparoscopic lavage or Hartman's procedure. The primary outcome was a composite endpoint of major morbidity and mortality within 12 months. Recruitment was terminated early after interim analysis of results demonstrated poorer outcomes in the laparoscopy group. At 30 days the combined primary outcome was 39% in the laparoscopic lavage group compared with 19% in the sigmoid colectomy group. Surgical re-interventions accounted for most of these adverse events. Follow-up continued to 12 months at which time the primary outcome measures were 60% and 67% between laparoscopic and open groups, respectively, with an OR of 1.28 (95% CI 0.54–3.03, p = 0.58) for the primary outcome in the laparoscopic lavage group. This includes 4 patients (9%) and 6 patients (14%) in the lavage and resection groups, respectively, who died during the study period (OR 0.53, 95% CI 0.13–2.15, p = 0.38) [41].

DILALA Study, a RCT from 9 centres in Sweden and Denmark, revealed findings in favour of laparoscopic lavage. In this study, 83 patients with purulent peritonitis at an initial diagnostic laparoscopy were randomised into laparoscopic lavage or Hartman's Procedure arms. The primary outcome of the study, reoperation rates at 12 months, is not yet reported, but short-term results at 3 months demonstrate similar rates of mortality (7.7 and 11.4%; p = 0.58) and reoperation rates (13.2 vs. 17.1%; p = 0.63) in lavage and resectional arms, respectively, while there was a shorter operation time, early recovery and less hospital stay in patients undergoing laparoscopic lavage [42].

Resection versus Conservative

The recently reported, MCRT "DIRECT" by Dutch investigators may provide stronger evidence in favour of resection. In this study, 109 patients with recurrent episodes (3 or more presentations in 2 years) or persistent abdominal complaints were allocated to sigmoid resection (ideally laparoscopic with primary anastomosis) or conservative management (intensive monitoring, lifestyle modification including supplementary dietary fibre, and analgesics or laxatives as required). Overall anastomotic leak rate was 12%. 21% received a stoma and at 6 months, 82% of stomas were reversed. However, study terminated early and recruited approximately half of the 214 participants stipulated by power calculations [43]. It has been previously documented that stopping such trials early, overestimates treatment effect, despite statistical compensation [44].

The Association of Coloproctologists of Great Britain and Ireland clearly differentiate between these indications for surgery and reject the need for universal elective resection [45]. This position is constant across age groups, as previously it was held that younger patients had a more virulent course.

Perforated Diverticulitis

In patients with diagnosis of acute diverticulitis, 1 to 2% of cases can develop perforation and the mortality is 20 - 30%. Hinchey Stage III (purulent peritonitis) and Hinchey Stage IV (free perforation with faecal peritonitis) are the main presentations for these variants. They require emergent operative intervention. One of the surgical options is Hartmann resection, but as already discussed 1/3rd will never undergo reversal. Resection with primary anastomosis is an alternative option and is superior to Hartmann in select patients with Hinchey III and IV. The decision to perform a particular procedure should be taken on case to case basis. Selected patients with purulent diverticulitis may be successfully treated by laparoscopic lavage without resection or at times may help to delay an emergent operation. The role still remains uncertain.

Fistulas

Fistulas occur in 2% of patients with diverticular disease. Colovesical fistula constitutes the commonest (65%) fistula. Colovesical Fistulas are more common in men. CT reveals air or contrast in bladder. Cystoscopy and colonoscopy should always be done to rule out a cancer. Treatment comprises of resection of affected segment with primary repair with interposition of omentum. Colovaginal fistula is usually seen in those patients of diverticulitis who have undergone a hysterectomy. Treatment is surgical which comprises of resection of affected segment with primary repair with interposition of omentum.

Diverticulitis with Abscess

Hinchey Stages I (pericolic abscess) and II (retroperitoneal or pelvic abscess) is seen in approximately 15% of patients with acute diverticulitis. They need admission plus intravenous antibiotics. Abscesses <2 cm should resolve on conservative treatment. Larger abscess are amenable to percutaneous drainage or at times elective resection [46].

Management of Acute Diverticulitis with Abscess after Drainage

Elective resection is typically advised after episode of complicated diverticulitis (ASCRS guidelines). Association of Colo-proctology of Great Britain and Ireland statement does not specifically address that and after percutaneous drainage of abscess, elective resection has been recommended as 41% will develop recurrence.

U. Minnesota group Gaertner et al. describe their 5-year experience with 218 patients treated with percutaneous drainage for diverticular abscess. At 7.4 year follow up, a majority of patients (85%) underwent colectomy, either emergently or electively and suggest nearly universal compliance with the 2006 Practice Parameters. In addition, the authors found that abscesses of >5cm were associated with emergency colectomies.

Diverticulitis with Obstruction

Obstruction can be partial or complete either due to oedema and/or inflammation. Recurrent attacks can cause inflammation and fibrosis resulting in stricture, which must be evaluated to rule out cancer.

Emergent Surgical Intervention

Anderson et al. [47] meta-analysis conducted a meta-analysis comparing the results of primary anastomosis (PA) with Hartmann procedure (HP). Total number of 50 studies were analysed which included 569 patients. Morbidity and mortality was found greater in HP group. The study concluded that PA is safer procedure than HP. They also concluded that PA with diverting loop ileostomy (DLI) in left sided perforation was safer, showed higher stoma reversal rate with less complications with shorter length of stay, and less patient expenditure.

Laparoscopic Resections

Sigma Trial, a multicenter double blind RCT laparoscopic versus open elective resection proved that laparoscopic and laparoscopic -assisted elective colon resections can be performed safely with low conversion and complication rates, with faster recovery, decreased length of stay, less postoperative pain and better cosmesis. Factors to be considered include body habitus, local tissue inflammation and complicated diverticulitis. More complicated disease may require conversion [48]. The late clinical outcomes did not differ between groups during the 30-day to 6-month follow-up period. Consideration of total postoperative morbidity shows a 27% reduction in major morbidity for patients undergoing laparoscopic surgery for diverticular disease. Laparoscopic versus Open prospective, multicenter, double-blind, parallel-arm, RCT in 5 centres showed a significantly more major complications in open group 9.6% vs. 25.0% ($P = 0.038$) along with less pain, improved quality of life, and shorter length of stay at the cost of a longer operating time. Minor complication rates were similar [49].

Laparoscopic Lavage is a new modality of treatment for perforated diverticulitis. This was first described by O'Sullivan et al. Ireland, who reported the results of 100 consecutive cases with 93% success (50). This concept is now catching up more and more with most of the surgeons because of increased adoption of laparoscopic surgery, improvement in CT imaging and advances in technical skill. Laparoscopic lavage has emerged as a promising therapeutic intervention. Overall intervention rate is same. Proportion of patients undergoing laparoscopic lavage has increased from 8% to 17%. Laparoscopic lavage is more likely a better option in patients at extremes of age.

Laparoscopic Lavage Systematic Review Publications 1990-2008

In this systematic review 8 studies met inclusion criteria and 213 patients with acute complicated diverticulitis were managed by laparoscopic lavage & antibiotics for Hinchey grade 3 disease. Conversion to laparotomy was made in 6 (3%) patients. Mean length of stay was 9 days. 10% had different types of complications. Mean follow up was 38 months. 38% underwent elective sigmoid resection with primary anastomosis as an alternative to more radical surgery in selected patients.

The SCANDIV trial, a multicentre randomised controlled trial involving 199 participants, randomised patients with suspected perforated diverticular disease to undergo either laparoscopic lavage or colonic resection. The primary endpoint was severe postoperative complications (defined as Clavien-Dindo complication of >IIIa) at 90 days. This was seen in 30.7% in the laparoscopic lavage group and 26.0% in the colon resection group (difference, 4.7% [95% CI –7.9 to 17.0]; $p = 0.53$), with a higher reoperation rate (12.9 vs. 8.3%) and 4 missed sigmoid cancers in the laparoscopic lavage group. The authors conclude that laparoscopic lavage does not reduce serious complication rates and has poorer secondary outcomes. For these reasons, they do not favour a laparoscopic lavage strategy [51].

Recurrence after Resection

Recurrent diverticulitis is rare after a colectomy for diverticulitis (3% to 13%). As many as 3% will require a redo resection. Thaler et al. found that level of anastomosis was the only predictor of recurrence. Important predictor is colo-sigmoid rather than colorectal anastomosis. Recurrence is 4 times more common in case of colo-sigmoid anastomosis. To avoid recurrences, the rectum should be used for anastomosis where taeina coli splay out onto upper rectum. [52].

CONCLUSION AND AGA GUIDELINES-2015

- Antibiotics should be used selectively in uncomplicated diverticulitis.
- Colonoscopy should be performed after resolution of acute diverticulitis.
- Prophylactic colonic resection in uncomplicated diverticulitis should be done on a case-by-case basis.
- A fiber-rich diet as well as physical activity is recommended after resolution.
- Aspirin use can be continued after resolution, particularly if it is being used for secondary prevention.
- It is not necessary to avoid nuts and popcorn in patients with diverticulosis or diverticulitis.
- Avoid non-aspirin, NSAIDs drugs if possible.
- Mesalamine, rifaximin, and probiotics are not recommended to prevent recurrence.
- Laparoscopy is likely to play a more prominent role even in the management of acute perforation.
- Few reports of successful management of Hinchey III and IV disease with laparoscopic peritoneal washout, plus colorrhaphy for perforation [53-55]. The results of these studies are quite promising.

- By delaying the elective operation the risks associated with Hartmann's procedure or primary anastomosis in a contaminated field can be avoided.
- This technique has been evaluated only in limited studies and is currently not part of the guidelines from ASCRS [56].
- Although the EAES has recommended that selected patients in selected centres be candidates for this procedure, they have not advocated this technique as a general recommendation [57].

REFERENCES

[1] Sandler, RS., Everhart, JE., Donowitz, M., Adams, E., Cronin, K., Goodman, C., etal.(May,2002) The burden of selected digestive diseases in the United States. *Gastroenterology*,122(5):1500-11.

[2] Stollman, N., Smalley, W. and Hirano, I. (Dec.2015). AGA Institute Clinical Guidelines Committee. American Gastroenterological Association Institute Guideline on the Management of Acute Diverticulitis. *Gastroenterology*, 149(7):1944-9.

[3] Morris, AM., Regenbogen, SE., Hardiman, KM. and Hendren S(2014). Sigmoid diverticulitis: a systematic review. *JAMA*, 311: 287–29.

[4] Jacobs DO.(2007). Clinical practice. Diverticulitis. *N Engl J Med*, 357: 2057–2066.

[5] Boostrom, SY., Wolff, BG., Cima, RR., Merchea, A., Dozois, EJ.and Larson DW(2012). Uncomplicated diverticulitis, more complicated than we thought. *J Gastrointest Surg,* 16: 1744–1749.

[6] Lau KC, Spilsbury K, Farooque Y, Kariyawasam SB, Owen RG, Wallace MH, et al. Is colonoscopy still mandatory after a CT diagnosis of left-sided diverticulitis: can colorectal cancer be confidently excluded? *Dis Colon Rectum*. 2011 Oct;54(10):1265-70.

[7] Swanson, SM., and Strate, LL(2018). Acute colonic diverticulitis. *Ann Intern Med*, 1: 168(9).

[8] Stollman, N., Smalley, W. and Hirano, I.(Dec.2015). AGA Institute Clinical Guidelines Committee. American Gastroenterological Association Institute Guideline on the Management of Acute Diverticulitis. *Gastroenterology*, 149(7):1944-9.

[9] Floch, MH (2006). A hypothesis: is diverticulitis a type of inflammatory bowel disease? *J Clin Gastroenterol*, 40(suppl 3): S121–S125.

[10] Tursi, A., Elisei, W., Brandimarte, G., Giorgetti, GM., Inchingolo, CD. and Nenna R, et al.(2012). Musosaltumour necrosis factor α in diverticular disease of the colon is overexpressed with disease severity. *Colorectal Dis*,14: e258–e263.

[11] Shabanzadeh, DM. and Wille-Jorgensen P(2012). Antibiotics for uncomplicated diverticulitis. *Cochrane Database Syst Rev*, 11: CD009092.

[12] Chabok, A., Påhlman, L., Hjern, F., Haapaniemi, S. and Smedh K(2012). AVOD Study Group: Randomized clinical trial of antibiotics in acute uncomplicated diverticulitis. *Br J Surg*, 99: 532–539.

[13] Daniels, L., Ünlü, Ç., de Korte, N., van Dieren, S., Stockmann, HB., Vrouenraets, BC, et al.(2017).Randomized clinical trial of observational versus antibiotic treatment for a first episode of CT-proven uncomplicated acute diverticulitis. *Br J Surg*, 104: 52–61.

[14] Shah, SD. and Cifu AS.(2017). Management of acute diverticulitis. *JAMA*,318: 291–292.

[15] Raskin, JB., Kamm, MA., Jamal, MM., Marquez, J., Melze,r E., Schoen, RE. et al. (2014). Mesalamine did not prevent recurrent diverticulitis in phase 3 controlled trials. *Gastroenterology*, 147: 793–802.

[16] Kruis, W., Kardalinos, V., Eisenbach. T., Lukas, M., Vich, T., Bunganic, I. et al. (2017). Randomised clinical trial: mesalazine versus placebo in the prevention of diverticulitis recurrence. *Aliment Pharmacol Ther*, 46: 282–291.

[17] Urushidani, S., Kuriyama, A. and Matsumura, M.(2018). 5-aminosalicylic acid agents for prevention of recurrent diverticulitis: a

systematic review and meta-analysis. *J Gastroenterol Hepatol*, 33: 12–19.

[18] Dughera, L., Serra, AM., Battaglia, E., Tibaudi, D., Navino, M. and Emanuelli. G.(2004). Acute recurrent diverticulitis is prevented by oral administration of a polybacterial lysate suspension. *Minerva Gastroenterol Dietol*, 50: 149–153.

[19] Bianchi, M., Festa, V., Moretti, A., Ciaco, A., Mangone, M. and Tornatore, V. et al. (2011). Meta-analysis: long-term therapy with rifaximin in the management of uncomplicated diverticular disease. *Aliment Pharmacol Ther,* 33: 902–910.

[20] Lahner, E., Bellisario, C., Hassan, C., Zullo, A., Esposito, G. and Annibale B.(2016). Probiotics in the treatment of diverticular disease. A systematic review. *J Gastrointestin Liver Dis,* 25: 79–86.

[21] Biondo, S., Golda, T., Kreisler, E., Espin, E., Vallribera, F., Oteiza, F. et al. (Jan, 2014). Outpatient versus hospitalization management for uncomplicated diverticulitis: a prospective, multicenter randomized clinical trial (DIVER Trial). *Ann Surg*, 259(1):38-44.

[22] Balasubramanian, I., Fleming, C., Mohan, HM., Schmidt, K., Haglind, E. and Winter, DC.(2017). Out-patient management of mild or uncomplicated diverticulitis: a systematic review. *Dig Surg*, 34: 151–160.

[23] Joliat, GR., Emery, J., Demartines, N., Hubner, M., Yersin, B., Hahnloser, D.(2017). Antibiotic treatment for uncomplicated and mild complicated diverticulitis: outpatient treatment for everyone. *Int J Colorectal Dis*, 32: 1313–1319.

[24] Feingold, D., Steele, SR. and Lee Sl. (March, 2014). Practice parameters for the treatment of sigmoid diverticulitis. *Dis Colon Rectum*, 57(3):284-94.

[25] Solomkin, JS., Mazuski, JE and Bradley JS.(Feb.2010). Diagnosis and management of complicated intra-abdominal infection in adults and children: guidelines by the Surgical Infection Society and the Infectious Diseases Society of America. *Surg Infect* (Larchmt). 11(1):79-109.

[26] Chapman J.(2005). Complicated diverticulitis: is it time to rethink the rules? *Ann Surg*, 242:576–581.

[27] Chapman JR.(2006).. Diverticulitis: a progressive disease? Do multiple recurrences predict less favorable outcomes? *Ann Surg*, 243:876–880.

[28] Deery, SE. and Hodin, RA. (Oct.2017). Management of Diverticulitis in 2017. *J Gastrointest Surg*,21(10): 1732–1741.

[29] Van'tSant, HP., Slieker, JC., Hop, WCJ., Weidema, WF., Lange, JF., Vermeulen, J. et al. (Aug. 2012). The influence of mechanical bowel preparation in elective colorectal surgery for diverticulitis. *Tech Coloproctol*, 16(4): 309–314.

[30] Klarenbeek, BR., Samuels, M., van der Wal, MA., van der Peet, DL., Meijerink, WJ. and Cuesta, MA.(April, 2010). Indications for elective sigmoid resection in diverticular disease. *Ann Surg*, 251(4):670-4.

[31] Hall, JF., Roberts, PL., Ricciardi, R., Read, T., Scheirey, C., Wald, C., Marcello, PW. and Schoetz, DJ. (March, 2011). Long-term follow-up after an initial episode of diverticulitis: what are the predictors of recurrence? *Dis Colon Rectum*, 54(3):283-8.

[32] Classen, JN., Bonardi, R., O'Mara, CS., Finney, DC. and Sterioff S.(Nov.1976).Surgical treatment of acute diverticulitis by staged procedures. *Ann Surg,* 184(5): 582–586.

[33] Cirocchi, R., Afshar, S., Di Saverio, S., Popivanov, G., De Sol, A., Gubbiotti, F, et al. (2017). A historical review of surgery for peritonitis secondary to acute colonic diverticulitis: from Lockhart-Mummery to evidence-based medicine. *World J Emerg Surg*,12: 14.

[34] Ince, M., Stocchi, L., Khomvilai, S., Kwon, DS., Hammel, JP. and Kiran, RP. (Aug. 2012). Morbidity and mortality of the Hartmann procedure for diverticular disease over 18 years in a single institution. *Colorectal Dis,* 14(8):e492-8.

[35] Banerjee, S., Leather, AJ., Rennie, JA., Samano, N., Gonzalez, JG. and Papagrigoriadis, S.(Sep. 2005). Feasibility and morbidity of reversal of Hartmann's. *Colorectal Dis,*7(5):454-9.

[36] Salem, L. and Flum, DR.(Nov. 2004). Primary anastomosis or Hartmann's procedure for patients with diverticular peritonitis? A systematic review. *Dis Colon Rectum*, 47(11):1953-64.

[37] Wong, WD., Wexner, SD., Lowry, A., Vernava 111, A., Burnstein, M., Dentsman F, et al. (2000). (Practice parameters for the treatment of sigmoid diverticulitis—Supporting documentation. *Dis Colon Rectum,* 43, 290–297 .

[38] Stollman, N., Smalley, W. and Hirano, I.(Dec.2015). *American Gastroenterological Association Institute Guideline on the Management of Acute Diverticulitis*, 14999 (7): 1944–1949.

[39] Van Arendonk, KJ., Tymitz, KM., Gearhart, SL., Stem. M. and Lidor, AO.(April.2013). Outcomes and costs of elective surgery for diverticular disease: a comparison with other diseases requiring colectomy. *JAMA Surg*, 148(4):316-21. doi: 10.1001/jamasurg.2013. 1010.

[40] Andeweg, CS., Berg, R., Staal, JB., ten Broek, RP. and van Goor, H.(Feb.2016). Patient-reported Outcomes After Conservative or Surgical Management of Recurrent and Chronic Complaints of Diverticulitis: Systematic Review and Meta-analysis. *Clin Gastroenterol Hepatol.* 14(2):183-90.

[41] Vennix, S., Musters, GD., Mulder, IM., Swank, HA., Consten, EC., Belgers, EH., et al. (2015). Laparoscopic peritoneal lavage or sigmoidectomy for perforated diverticulitis with purulent peritonitis: a multicentre, parallel-group, randomised, open-label trial. *Lancet,* 386: 1269–1277.

[42] Thornell, A., Angenete, E., Gonzales, E., Heath, J., Jess, P., Lackberg, Z., et al.(2011). Treatment of acute diverticulitis laparoscopic lavage vs. resection (DILALA): study protocol for a randomised controlled trial. *Trials,*12: 186.

[43] Stam, V, MAW., Draaisma, WA., Stellato, R., Bemelman, WA., Boermeester, MA. et al. (Jan.2017). Surgery versus conservative management for recurrent and ongoing left-sided diverticulitis (DIRECT trial): an open-label, multicentre, randomised controlled trial. *Lancet Gastroenterol Hepatol,* 2(1):13-22.

[44] Bassler, D., Briel, M., Montori, VM., Lane, M., Glasziou, P., Zhou, Q, et al. (March,2010). Stopping randomized trials early for benefit and estimation of treatment effects: systematic review and meta-regression analysis. *JAMA*, 24;303(12):1180-7.

[45] Fozard, JB1., Armitage, NC., Schofield, JB. and Jones, OM.(2011). ACPGBI position statement on elective resection for diverticulitis. *Colorectal Dis*,13: 1–11.

[46] Rafferty, J., Shellito, P., Hyman, NH. and Buie, WD.(July,2006). Standards Committee of American Society of Colon and Rectal Surgeons. Practice parameters for sigmoid diverticulitis. *Dis Colon Rectum*, 49 (7):939-44.

[47] Anderson, BA., Salem, L. and Flum, DR.(Sep.2005). A systematic review of whether oral contrast is necessary for the computed tomography diagnosis of appendicitis in adults. *Am J Surg*, 190(3):4.

[48] Klarenbeek, BR., Veenhof, AA., Bergamaschi, R., van der Peet, DL., van den Broek, WT., de Lange, ES., et al. (Jan.2009). Laparoscopic sigmoid resection for diverticulitis decreases major morbidity rates: a randomized control trial: short-term results of the Sigma Trial. *Ann Surg*, 249(1):39-44.

[49] Teeuwen, PH., chouten, MG., Bremers, AJ. and Bleichrodt, RP.(Sep.2009). Laparoscopic sigmoid resection for diverticulitis decreases major morbidity rates: a randomized controlled trial. *Ann Surg*,250(3):500-1; author reply 501-2.

[50] O'Sullivan, GC., Murphy, D., O'Brien, MG. and Ireland A.(April, 1996). Laparoscopic management of generalized peritonitis due to perforated colonic diverticula. *Am J Surg*, 171(4):432-4.

[51] Schultz, JK., Yaqub, S., Wallon, C., Blecic, L., Forsmo, HM., Folkesson, J, et al.(2015). Laparoscopic lavage vs primary resection for acute perforated diverticulitis: the SCANDIV randomized clinical trial. *JAMA*, 314: 1364–1375.

[52] Thaler, K., Baig, MK., Berho, M., Weiss, EG., Nogueras, JJ., Arnaud, JP., et al.(Mar.2003). Determinants of recurrence after sigmoid resection for uncomplicated diverticulitis. *Dis Colon Rectum*, 46(3): 385-8.

[53] Ricciardi, R., Baxter, NN., Read, TE., Marcello, PW., Hall, J. and Roberts PL.(Sep.2009). Is the decline in the surgical treatment for diverticulitis associated with an increase in complicated diverticulitis? *Dis Colon Rectum*, 52(9):1558-63.

[54] Mutter, D., Bouras, G., Forgione, A., Vix, M., Leroy, J. and Marescaux, J.(Jul,2006). Two-stage totally minimally invasive approach for acute complicated diverticulitis. *Colorectal Dis,* 8(6):501-5.

[55] Franklin, ME Jr., Jacobs, M. and Plasencia, G.(1997). Laproscopic surgery applicable to complicated colonic diverticular disease? *Surg Endosc*, 11(10):1021-1025.

[56] Santaniello, M. and Bergamaschi, R. (Jul,2007). Perforated diverticulitis: should the method of surgical access to the abdomen determine treatment? *Colorectal Dis*, 9(6):494-5.

[57] Sauerland, S., Agresta, F., Bergamaschi, R., Borzellino, G., Budzynski, A., Champault, G., et al. (Jan.2006). Laparoscopy for abdominal emergencies: evidence-based guidelines of the European Association for Endoscopic Surgery. *Surg Endosc*,20(1):14-29. Epub 2005 Oct 24.

About the Authors

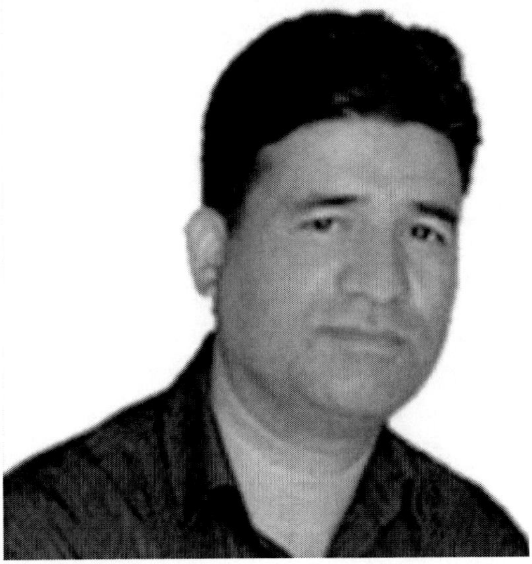

Shams ul Bari completed his postgraduate training in General surgery at Sher-i-Kashmir Institute of Medical Sciences (SKIMS), Srinagar, India. He is presently working as an Associate Professor in the Department of Surgery, SKIMS Medical College, Srinagar Kashmir. Earlier, he worked as a consultant at Government Gousia Hospital, Srinagar Kashmir. He is a fellow of International college of surgeons (FICS) and Indian Association of Gastrointestinal Endoscopic Surgeons (FIAGES) . He has more than 70 publications to his credit published in various national and international journals. He has contributed book chapters in several international books of repute. He has also authored a book entitled, Human Abdominal Hydatidosis, published by Springer. He serves on the editorial board of several international journals including *World Journal of Gastroenterology* and *World Journal of Gastrointestinal Surgery*.

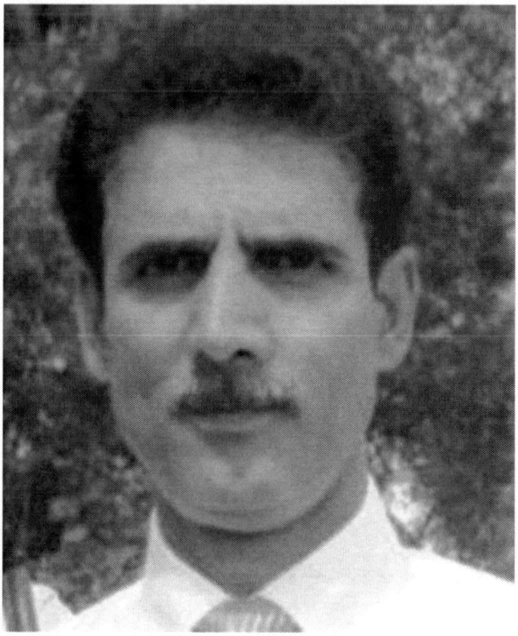

Ajaz Ahmad Malik completed his postgraduate training in general surgery at Sher-i-Kashmir Institute of Medical Sciences (SKIMS), Srinagar, India, which he subsequently joined as a faculty member. He is presently working as Professor and division head at the Department of General and Minimal Invasive Surgery, SKIMS.He is a fellow of the International College of Surgeons (FICS), Indian Association of Gastrointestinal Endoscopic Surgeons (FIAGES) and an associate fellow of the American College of Surgeons (FACS). . He has more than 80 research papers, published in various national and international journals He has also several book chapters to his credit. He is one of the authors of the book entitled, Human Abdominal Hydatidosis, published by Springer .

INDEX

B

C

D

E

F

G

H

I

J

K

L

M

N

O

P

Q

R

S

T

U

V

W